DI

Before you start any new supplement program consult with your doctor, especially if you are under a doctor's care, are using drugs, are pregnant, or have a serious illness. The author disclaim responsibility for any adverse effects or unforeseen consequences resulting from the use of this product and information contained in this book.

The information in this book is not intended as medical advice, to diagnose, treat, cure and prevent any disease. This type of medical advice should be obtained from your doctor. The U.S. FDA has not approved this product. Consult your doctor when using new remedies or techniques when dealing with various illness or symptoms.

The Diva's Guide to an Acne-Free Life

One Girl's Journey from Zitty to Pretty

Dawn Amador

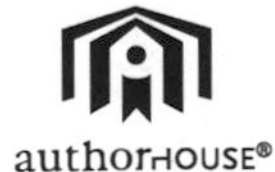

AuthorHouse™
1663 Liberty Drive
Bloomington, IN 47403
www.authorhouse.com
Phone: 1-800-839-8640

Published by AuthorHouse 07/19/2012

ISBN: 978-1-4772-0699-7 (sc)
ISBN: 978-1-4772-0700-0 (e)

Library of Congress Control Number: 2012908686

This book is printed on acid-free paper.

To my sons, Anatol and Andrzej.

You have given me the greatest gifts life has to offer: joy, laughter, and unconditional love.

Acknowledgments

I thank Erin Finot for her love and friendship—thank you for not being able say no to me. I am grateful to my mother for teaching me the virtue of perseverance. Dr. Bryce Renshaw, thank you for your support. Lisbeth Boger of Éminence Organic Skin Care. Shelly Hancock of Real Transformation Center. To the dedicated staff at Skin Inc. Magazine. Christine and Vanessa for your emotional support. To my clients who let me into their lives; without you, there would not be a book.

I would like to thank Tim Tabke at Phoenix Productions, Raymond Rodriguez for my cover photo, Lauren Eaton for my hair and Tiffany Galace for my makeup. Last, to IJ; you forever altered my universe.

TABLE OF CONTENTS

Foreword

Since the first publication of my book I have changed some things in my life. I have been on a spiritual path of mindfulness and meditation for almost three years now. My journey inward has changed me in many ways, and one specific change that has taken place in my life is my choice to become a raw foodist. What does this mean? Simply put I eat almost all my food raw, and I abstain from all animal flesh.

What was the catalyst for this change? I found the more I meditated the less I craved meat and cooked food. It also just seemed like a kinder way to traverse though the planet. I did not make this change over night. I never believe in extremes. I feel when we are extreme with our bodies and mind we become unbalanced. My journey into becoming a raw foodist was a gradual and slow progression. I started off changing my diet to fifty percent raw, and over the time span of a year I become almost one hundred percent raw.

I woke up one morning, and I had zero desire to eat cooked food or animal protein. I am not advocating that eating animal protein is wrong. I have many friends who eat meat. I just always encourage them to choose sustainable organic meat over factory-produced meat. Therefore, I intend to keep all my recipes in the book that are cooked or meat based, but I will also add some raw options for those of you who want to join me on this journey of living raw.

You can also follow me on YouTube for updated recipes and tutorials on living raw. I always test every recipe on my seven and five year old sons. I figured if they like it almost everyone would. Go to my website www.skinlogic.us and click on my YouTube channel. If you have any specific recipe you would like to see let me know!

Introduction

If you met me as a child, you would never guess I would grow into a woman who is passionate about everything fashion and skin care. You see I grew up on the back of a hay lot in Chino, California to an extremely poor family.

As a child, I worried more about basics necessities such as food and shelter than I cared about fashion and skin care. Honestly, I do not remember my mother cleansing her skin beyond occasionally rubbing vegetable oil on it. We were definitely too poor to worry about fashion.

In my dysfunctional surroundings, I do not recall thinking much about being a girl and what it entailed. While most girls dreamed of pink and fairytales, I dreamed of a life away from the daily violence of my home life. I dreamed of having an emotionally available mother; to feel safe and comforted. So, I did exactly that; I started dreaming day and night.

My dreams and fantasies for a better life came through reading books. At a very young age, I started to lose myself in books. I would read and dream of far away places, girls dressing up for tea parties with their friends, and perfect families sitting around the dinner table sharing a meal.

As I grew older, and my reading vocabulary expanded, I read and dreamed about fashion and beautiful things. I remember picking up my first issue of *Vogue*. As I flipped through the pages, it appeared to be a strange, mystical world full of beautiful and exotic things. I was mesmerized and captivated.

I visited local grocery stores and clothing outlets, strolling up and down the aisles to look at the beautiful palettes of makeup. I would visualize my spectacular transformation using the beautiful color palettes. I walked the clothing aisles, touching fabrics and running them through my fingers. It felt blissful, yet it was agonizing. I longed to put the beautiful colors on my face, and feel the lustrous fabrics on my body. These outing were heavenly and torturous.

By the age of twelve, my father was sent to prison; my family went to live with my grandfather in Whittier, California. At the time, Whittier seemed like a cosmopolitan city compared to being on the back of a hay lot in Chino, California.

The first chance I got, I hopped on the bus and went to the Whittwood Mall. I will never forget the first time I walked through the mall entrance. It may as well have been Fifth Avenue in New York City. All the stores hypnotized me.

I ended up in Macy's and was taken by all the makeup counters and skin care bottles. I walked up to the Estée Lauder counter, and asked the saleswoman, "What's in the bottles?" She looked at me as if I had just arrived into the twentieth century.

Though she knew she was not going to get a sale from me, she still walked me through each skin care program Estée Lauder had to offer—I was in heaven! I climbed back on the bus, dreaming of the Estée Lauder Skin Care System the entire way home.

A few months later, my grandfather died and left my mother some money. Knowing her children had grown up with so little, my mother offered to take us out individually to experience a special day with her. When my day arrived, I knew exactly where I wanted to go—Macy's!

I had been dreaming of this day ever since that bus ride home. Walking into Macy's that day, I felt like a million bucks. I marched over to the saleswoman and asked her for the Estée Lauder Skin Care System; it even came with an exfoliating brush!

I was so excited; I went home that night and methodically went through my new regime. I will never forget the smells and feeling of the fluids applied to my face. I was forever changed. For the first time in my life,

I felt special and beautiful—part of some secret circle of women I had only seen in magazines.

That Estée Lauder Skin Care System may as well have been gold. I cherished and reverenced those bottles like they were the most valuable artifacts in the world. It was in those moments, my love for skin care began.

Luckily, I had flawless skin throughout my teenage years. However, in my twenties, my skin took revenge on me—my battle with acne started. I became so obsessed with wanting clear skin again; some would say it took over my life.

In my desire for acne-free skin, I have basically read every skin care and nutrition book published, tried nearly every remedy suggested, and tested every product invented. I even invented homemade products, which I diligently tested on any willing friend.

So, join me on my journey—a culmination of tireless research and true passion to live a happy, acne-free life.

With love and beauty,

Dawn

CHAPTER 1

What is Acne?

I know one thing for sure: acne sucks. I hated my skin and face when I looked into the mirror; I saw cysts and discoloration all over. I detested the way acne made me feel about myself; it robbed me of my self-confidence.

I wanted to scrub my face off; hoping if I scrubbed hard enough, the acne would go away. I despised when these inflamed lesions depressed me, making me want to hide from the world. At times, I felt so awful I would walk into a room with my head down, or buried in a turtleneck to hide as much of my face as possible, because I felt so ugly.

There were times when I cried myself to sleep. I would pray whatever cream or potion I was currently using would convert my skin complexion into perfection by morning—my prayers for perfect skin never did manifest.

My tears turned into frustration and self-hatred. I despised my skin and figured I had to live my adult life with ugly lesions randomly popping up all over my face.

That is, until one day when I decided I did not care if I had to make nurturing clear skin a career. Whatever it took, one day I would be rid of the ugly lesions, which scarred and disfigured my face.

What exactly is acne? It is a disease onset by dead skin cells combining with oil, resulting in a blockage of the pore or sebaceous gland. When the sebaceous gland is filled with blackheads, inflamed papules, pustules, inflamed nodules, and cysts, we experience acne. The causes of acne can be numerous. That is, acne can be caused by hormone imbalances, diet, stress, and other lifestyle choices.

When acne is present, sebum production, as well as bacterial colonization, is abnormal. It should be noted; everyone has propionibacterium acnes (p. acne) bacteria, which lives in the sebaceous glands.

P. Acne bacteria become a problem when the normal process of cellular turnover is compromised causing the dead skin cells to not shed from the follicle. These cells trap oil in the follicle and the p. acne bacteria feed off the oil and excrete the by-product of inflammatory, toxic, and corrosive fatty acids.

In turn, abnormal colonization of bacteria causes an inflammatory response by the chemical breakdown of oils and fats within our clogged sebaceous gland. When blackheads (bacteria and debris) within our pores become inflamed, the walls within the pore rupture and release cellular and lipid (oil) material into the dermis.

This process causes an inflammatory response and cysts are born. Those lovely white-yellowish inflamed acnes are the aftermath of the war our immune system waged to combat inflammation within the pore.

CHAPTER 2

Diet and Acne

Let food be thy medicine, thy medicine shall be thy food.

—Hippocrates

In my twenties I was plagued with a horrible skin disease—acne. I was so perplexed with why my skin suddenly turned on me. I literally had flawless skin up to that point. Ever since the day I brought home my first skin care products, I had been diligent about taking care of my face.

I was eating healthier than I ever had because as a child, I ate boxed food from food banks, old cuts of meat, and endless fast food meals. So, why, when I was living in Northern California—the mecca of organic food and farmers markets—was my skin breaking out in cystic acne?

All I knew for certain: my self-esteem was dropping by the second. I was making matters worse by applying endless layers of foundation to my face in an attempt to cover my acne.

In an attempt to clear my skin, I started experimenting with different types of diets. I would try a high protein diet followed by a vegan diet, followed by some hybrid vegetarian diet. Naturally, I began to think all my experimentation with food may have been the culprit.

I decided to stick to a quasi-vegan diet for a while to see if it would help. It did not. In fact, my acne became worse. On top of that, I was starting to get scars and discoloration was developing all over my face.

I felt helpless and depressed then upon reading *The Clear Skin Prescription*, by Dr. Perricone, I started to look at acne in a whole new light. At length, Dr. Perricone discusses how acne is an inflammatory disease, and anyone suffering from it should avoid foods that cause inflammation in the system.

Why does food cause inflammation? Well, if a person has an allergic reaction to something ingested, his or her body has an inflammatory response in order to protect it. In turn, the immune system mistakes the body's normal healthy tissue as an invader and attacks it.

If a person continues to eat foods that cause this response, then he or she is putting his or her body in a state of chronic inflammation. After some time, this can cause a host of problems that impact quality of life.

The main foods that cause inflammation are pretty much those, which make eating, fun and exciting. Seriously, think of any carbohydrate, and then imagine never eating it again, or at least only on rare occasions.

Yes, most carbohydrates cause blood sugar to spike, which, in turn, causes inflammation in the system. Why do carbohydrates, especially high-glycemic carbohydrates create an inflammatory response within the system? When large quantities of pasta, high sugary sweets, and baked goods hit the system, they convert into sugar once they enter the bloodstream. The high levels of sugar now present in the system throws blood sugar levels out of balance. To bring blood sugar levels back into balance the pancreas responds by upping insulin in the bloodstream to bring blood sugar levels back into homeostasis. This is an important function because high levels of blood sugar in the system create chemical reactions, which causes inflammation that leads to free radical damage within the cell. Free radical damage within the cell can lead to the onset of acne, or exacerbate existing acne conditions as well as cause a host of other problems.

The other downside of the body being barraged by a high intake of high-glyclimic foods is that it is constantly trying to stabilize blood sugar levels. If there is a constant stream of high-glycemic foods entering the system the pancreas becomes overworked, and over time it has difficulty bringing blood sugar levels back to normal—leading to larger problems such as diabetes, obesity, and accelerated aging.

Desperately wanting clear and healthy skin, I tried the Perricone Diet, which consists of eating a lot of oatmeal, blueberries, and salmon. Trust me, I did not develop a natural pallet for fish; remember, I grew up on boxed food and red meat.

I tried to follow this diet on and off again for months; it was excruciating. I am not a big breakfast eater either, so having to down bowls of oatmeal every morning was extremely difficult for me.

Also, I do not care much for salmon. However, I try to like it; convincing myself it is amazing for me. Although, I always ended up drowning it in butter. I frustratingly felt like I was taking one step forward and two steps back trying to maintain this diet. That is, butter as well as other dairy products can be detrimental for those of us suffering from acne conditions. I was therefore negating most of the beneficial effects of eating salmon.

So, with all the well-intentions in the world, I knew I could not maintain this diet long-term if I wanted to remain sane.

Chapter 3

The Alkaline Principle

There was not much improvement in my skin condition anyway since I could not remain consistent on the Perricone diet, so I stopped torturing myself with sporadic meals of oatmeal and salmon. Next, I learned about Bragg® Apple Cider Vinegar (ACV) and started diligently drinking the following ACV cocktail, which consisted of:

- 2 tsp. apple cider vinegar
- 1 tsp. honey
- 1 tsp. cayenne pepper
- A small amount of warm water

Drink this mixture three times a day to detoxify the body; subsequently, improving skin health. Today, I only take ACV once a day, adding one teaspoon of cayenne pepper. The value in ACV: it is alkaline in nature.

What does it mean for something to be alkaline? An integral component of the body and the optimal functioning of body tissue is for it to have a proper balance of alkaline and acidity. Remember the pH scale from science class? In chemistry, the pH stands for potential hydrogen. On the pH scale: 0.0 = completely acidic, 7.0 = completely neutral, and 14.0 = completely alkaline.

Studies show proper blood pH should be in the pH 7.3 range. However, as a result of our modern diet of processed foods and sugary drinks, most of our food consumption is on the acidic range of the scale.

The modern diet is laden with foods that leave an acidic residue in the bloodstream, rather than an alkaline. The trouble occurs when our bodies go into acid overload and start leaching minerals out of our tissues in order to maintain a proper pH level.

Why is it a problem? When the body does not have the proper balance of minerals, the body's detoxification pathways can be hindered by this imbalance. When our capability to detoxify becomes impeded, toxic sludge starts building up in our system, leading the way to disease and inflammation. This can result in acne, obesity, and a plethora of other inflammatory diseases.

So, how do we avoid the over acidification of our bodies? For starters, Bragg® ACV is high in trace minerals, especially potassium. It can aid in bringing the body back into a more alkaline state. Eating mineral rich foods can also aid in bringing the body back into balance.

The following is a list of alkaline and acidic foods that can balance the body and reduce inflammation:

ALKALINE FOODS	ACIDIC FOODS
ALKALIZING VEGETABLES:	**ACIDIFYING VEGETABLES:**
Alfalfa	Corn
Beets	Lentils
Broccoli	Olives
Cabbage	**ACIDIFYING FRUITS:**
Carrot	Blueberries
Cauliflower	Cranberries
Celery	Currants
Chlorella	Plums**
Cucumber	Prunes**
Dandelions	**ACIDIFYING GRAINS:**
Dulce	Amaranth
Eggplant	Barley
Garlic	Bran
Kale	Bread
Kohlrabi	Corn
Lettuce	Cornstarch
Mushrooms	Crackers,

ALKALINE FOODS	ACIDIC FOODS
Nightshade Veggies	Kamut
Onions	Macaroni
Peas	Noodles
Peppers	Oatmeal
Pumpkin	Quinoa
Radishes	Rye
Rutabaga	Spaghetti
Spinach	Spelt
Spirulina	Wheat
Sprouts	**ACIDIFYING DAIRY:**
Tomatoes	Butter
Watercress	Cheese
ALKALIZING ORIENTAL VEGETABLES:	**ACIDIFYING NUTS & BUTTERS:**
Daikon	Cashews
Kombu	Legumes
Maitake	Peanuts
Nori	Pecans

ALKALINE FOODS	**ACIDIC FOODS**
Reishi	Tahini
Shitake	Walnuts
Umebosh	**ACIDIFYING ANIMAL PROTEIN:**
Wakame	Bacon
ALKALIZING FRUITS:	Beef
Apple	Carp
Apricot	Clams
Avocado	Cod
Banana	Fish
Blackberries	Haddock
Cantaloupe	Lamb
Cherries	Lobster
Coconut	Mussels
Currants	Oyster
Grapes	Pike
Grapefruit	Pork
Lemon	Rabbit
Lime	Salmon

ALKALINE FOODS	ACIDIC FOODS
Muskmelons	Sardines
Nectarine	Sausage
Orange	Scallops
Peach	Shellfish
Pear	Shrimp
Pineapple	Tuna
Raisins	Turkey
Raspberries	Veal
Rhubarb	**SWEETENERS:**
Strawberries	Carob
Tangerine	Sugar
Tomato	**ACIDIFYING ALCOHOL:**
Watermelon	Beer
ALKALIZING PROTEIN:	Spirits
Almonds	Wine
Chestnuts	**ACIDIFYING:**
Millet	Catsup
Tempeh (fermented)	Cocoa

ALKALINE FOODS	ACIDIC FOODS
ALKALIZING SWEETENERS:	Coffee
Stevia	Mustard
ALKALIZING SPICES & SEASONINGS:	Pepper
Cinnamon	Vinegar
Curry	**CHEMICALS:**
Ginger	Drugs, Psychedelic
Herbs (all)	Herbicides
Miso	Pesticides
Mustard	Tobacco
Tamari	
ALKALIZING MINERALS:	
Calcium=pH12	
Cesium-pH14	
Magnesium=pH9	
Potassium=pH14	
Sodium=pH14	

Ever since I learned about the impact of acidic and alkaline foods on the body, I have diligently tried to consume as many foods on the alkaline chart as possible. I find when I focus on an alkaline diet I feel better and have more energy.

Everything But The Kitchen Sink Alkalinizing Salad

Throw all your favorite fruits and veggies over a bed of mixed greens.

Dressing

- 2 tbsp. of olive oil
- 2 tbsp. of apple cider vinegar
- 1 tsp. ground pepper

Clear Skin Tonic

- 8 oz of water
- 2 tbsp. of apple cider vinegar
- 4 mint leaves
- squeeze of lime

Drink this tonic everyday to help alkalinize the body and clear the skin.

CHAPTER 4

The Dark Side of Gluten

There I was trying to eat as healthy as possible, yet my skin continued breaking out. I will admit my acne was much better than it had been in previous years, but I did not have flawless skin all girls dream about.

Then one day I was chatting with a woman at a conference I attended in Las Vegas. She asked me if I had gluten in my diet. Gluten? I had no idea what gluten was at the time. So, when I got back home, I researched gluten and its connection to acne.

Gluten is a protein found primarily in wheat, oats, barley, and rye. People, who cannot tolerate gluten, have an autoimmune response in the small intestine, which may cause inflammation in the intestinal track.

The medical term for gluten intolerance is celiac disease. Celiac disease may cause a host of health problems such as digestive problems, depression, acne, and gallstones to name a few. The only way to reverse the effects of gluten is to eliminate it from one's diet.

My initial response: everything I love contains gluten. At first, when I decided to go gluten-free, I thought: *What am I going to eat?*

I was used to supplementing my diet with protein bars and cereal when I was insanely busy with life, work, and motherhood. So, how was I going to make it through hectic days while maintaining a gluten-free diet?

Well, I had to get creative and come up with quick, easy ways to incorporate gluten-free foods with minimal prep time into my diet. I began baking batches of roughly ten chicken breasts and yams, throwing them into individual containers to quickly grab in the mornings as I whisked myself and my two sons off into the world. I also made various smoothies and always made certain to carry handfuls of nuts with me.

About a month into my gluten-free diet, amazing things started to happen. My tendency was to wake up each morning in a fog, downing several cups of black tea in order to function. Well, the fogginess started to lift. I also experienced more energy throughout the day, even though my sleep habits had not changed much. My afternoon slumps, when I had to head to the local coffee shop, also dissipated. Additionally, the mid-day headache I chronically experienced vanished. Life seemed a little less jet-lagged.

In general, I felt happier and more optimistic in my daily life. My skin also started to improve. The deep cysts, which formed around my jaw line during my menstrual cycle, disappeared.

My skin developed a deep glow it had never emitted before. Even when I was a teenager, I did not have the healthy glow I lusted after. I always felt it was some sort of a tradeoff—to have either clear, dehydrated, flat skin, or blemished, oily skin.

I strived for the former, but longed for a clear, dewy look. Who wants to duck underneath a desk throughout the day to blot excessive oil from her skin? This routine is not so hot when one is crushing on the cute guy in the next cubical, right?

My life and skin were dramatically improving because of a gluten-free diet. The diet was not as bad as I had anticipated; within a few weeks, my cravings for bread and baked goods completely disappeared. I craved less sugar and my glycemic levels stabilized, relieving me of that feeling of energy and joy after eating starchy and sweet foods only to crash a few hours later.

In general, life was on the upswing and amazing things started to transpire. People were actually stopping me on the street to tell me how amazing my skin looked. Initially, I had to confirm they were referring to me, then as I walked, thought: *Yeah, me!*

I was finally becoming the girl with the amazing skin. It transformed my life and self-esteem.

CHAPTER 5

Why is Dairy So Evil?

Dairy is one of the main culprits to trigger inflammation in the system. Again, this is caused by the body's immune response to dairy, causing it to produce inflammation to protect itself.

Also, dairy products are acidic, can be difficult to digest, can cause inflammation, and cause insulin levels to rise. An inflammatory response from dairy can occur within the system if you have a dairy allergy. The inflammation response is caused by your body identifying the proteins in dairy as dangerous to the system. Your body then produces histamine, E antibodies and a host of other chemicals to attack the allergen. As well as possibly causing inflammation, dairy naturally raises insulin levels and insulin-like growth homrmone-1. When insulin levels are raised it triggers the male hormone androgen. When you overproduce the androgen hormone the male hormone receptors open up and trigger the acne process. An easy way to find out if dairy is a trigger or a cause of acne or other symptoms is to eliminate it for a few weeks to see if acne or other symptoms disappear.

Now, I know when I consume most dairy products, I must up the ante on my skin care routine to attack unwanted invaders. If I fail to do so, I usually experience a few unwanted visitors lurking on my cheek area.

Another big offender is sugar—consuming it causes a rapid rise in blood sugar, which like dairy causes an insulin response, which then causes an inflammatory response. If we continually eat foods, which cause spikes in blood sugar, our bodies have constant inflammation at a cellular level.

Constant inflammation in the body taxes the immune system. It can lead to inflammatory diseases such as cancer, arthritis, and acne. Even though acne is not a disease known to cause death if untreated, it can contribute to the death to one's self-esteem and social life.

Therefore, eliminating foods that cause inflammation and insulin spikes is imperative to controlling acne, as well as protecting ourselves from an onslaught of other inflammatory diseases. We can not only control our insulin levels by eating foods packed with amazing antioxidants, but also control and possibly negate the inflammatory response within our system.

What foods help battle against inflammation in the system? Well, pretty much everything on the aforementioned alkaline list. That is, most non-processed fruits, vegetables, and lean meats.

How do we get started on this meal plan to unleash beautiful skin and our inner diva? First, we need to clean out our cupboards and refrigerators of anything, which may block us from reaching diva status.

Before we go shopping, we need to get the largest trash bag available and rid our kitchen and lives of what is keeping us from being our most healthy beautiful selves. This purging includes all boxed, processed, and dairy-laden foods. Now, let's go shopping.

CHAPTER 6

Simple, Mind-Blowing, Anti-Inflammatory Meals

I strive to have 50 percent of my diet consist of raw foods, so we will consider some amazing smoothie recipes. This first smoothie is hands-down my favorite. When I am traveling and do not drink it for a few days, my body goes into withdrawals.

By the way, I do not measure portions. Simply throw a little of this and that, but for the sake of those who love measuring cups, I have listed quantities:

The Most Amazing Smoothie Ever

- 1 banana
- 1 apple
- 1 pear
- ½ lemon juice
- 2 cups of frozen mixed berries (Costco's organic antioxidant mix)
- ½ cup acai juice
- ½ cup pomegranate juice
- ½ cup of aloe vera juice
- 3 stalks of celery
- ¼ cup parsley
- ½ cucumber
- 2 cups of kale
- 3 cups of spinach
- 3 cups of mixed greens
- ½ raw beets
- 1 tbsp. of maca root
- ½ cup of raw vanilla flavored hemp powder

First, pour all the juices into a high quality blender and then add the mixed greens, spinach, and frozen fruit. Next, add everything else to super charge your immune system with an amazing cocktail of antioxidant super powers!

Please note, a high quality blender is really necessary; there are several out there on the market; do some research. They are fairly expensive, but deals can be found; they are totally worth the investment.

This recipe makes about seventy-two ounces of the most amazing smoothie ever. This is one day's worth of smoothies, which can be conveniently stored in spill-proof blender bottles to carry around throughout the day.

This next smoothie I love to drink pre—and post-workout is:

Almond Coconut Delight

- ¼ cup of almond butter
- 2 tbs. of virgin coconut oil
- 2 bananas
- 1 cup chocolate hemp powder
- 1 tbsp. of cinnamon
- 12 oz. of coconut milk

This recipe yields about twenty ounces; simply throw it all into the blender and mix. I drink ten ounces before a workout and ten ounces afterwards.

Glowing Skin Smoothie

- 8 oz. carrot juice
- 1 chunk of fresh ginger
- 1 cup frozen peaches
- 1 apple

Carrot juice is very high in vitamin A and ginger is an excellent anti-inflammatory, so drinking this smoothie on a regular basis really brings a nice glow to the skin.

This next smoothie is really satisfying when I crave something sweet and fluffy. I usually do not take in much dairy, but I do put whey powder in this smoothie as it gives it a nice whip cream texture.

Strawberry Dream Smoothie

- 1 cup frozen strawberries
- 1 ripe banana
- 8 oz. coconut milk
- ½ lemon (squeeze juice into blender)
- 2 scoops of vanilla whey protein powder
- 1 packet of stevia

Strawberries have very high water content, so they keep the skin hydrated and glowing. They are also high in salicylic acid; therefore, rubbing the remaining strawberries on the face creates a nice glow.

I drink smoothies or juices during the first half of the day. Our cells are primed to absorb more nutrients this way; especially, when the digestive system is not laden with heavy foods and proteins. Also, when we awaken, our bodies are still in detoxification mode from the night before. Our digestive system is not yet overloaded by digesting heavy proteins.

The more time we feed our bodies to detoxify and cleanse, the more likely we are to lower inflammation and have less toxic buildup in our bodies. This also means more time our bodies have to absorb a powerhouse of anti-inflammatory agents to help heal our cells and clear problematic skin.

After many grams of blissful smoothie perfection, I move onto nourishing, but less readily digestible foods. I generally snack on nuts, trail mix, and sweet potato bites, which I love. My recipe is as follows:

Get Your Glow On Morning Elixir

I love making this juice when I get up in the morning. It is packed full of antioxidant energy.

- 2 apples
- 4 stocks of celery
- ½ beet plus the leafy greens
- ½ lime (leave the peel on)
- 3 1-inch slices of daikon radish.

The benefits of this juice are: beets and lime (or lemon) are great hormone regulators, daikon radish is a wonderful liver cleanser, celery is high in vitamin C, and the phytonutrients in apples can help regulate blood sugar.

Purify Me

- 3 apples
- 6 dandelion leaves
- 1 cucumber (skin on)
- 1 head of butter lettuce
- 1 tbsp fresh ginger

Ginger is anti-inflammatory, and the benefits of dandelion are astounding. The healing properties of dandelion that are standouts for acne suffers are: anti-inflammatory, blood purifier, and may help in healing various skin conditions such as acne.

Get creative with juicing. I go to the Farmer's Market every week and add different fruits and vegetables to my juices. Also, if you have fresh juices in the morning have it before your smoothie. It is best for your digestive system to go from the most easily digestible foods to foods that take longer to digest.

An example of this would be: juice, smoothie, salad, chia seed pudding, heavier raw or cook proteins. I tend to keep my diet really simple. If you would like to uncook some more extravagant raw food meals on special occasions there are many fantastic raw food cookbooks on the market.

Fresh Almond Milk

I found it difficult adjusting to nut milks when I was initially trying to eliminate dairy from my diet. Then I started making my own fresh almond milk every morning, and I have never looked back. Fresh almond milk is sweet, creamy, and delicious.

Soak one cup of raw almonds in purified water overnight. In the morning drain the water, and put the almonds into the blender with three cups of purified water (I use the NURTiBULLET™).

Strain the almond milk through a nut milk bag or cheesecloth. You can find nut milk bags at most health food stores. Once the almond milk is strained pour it back in the blender with two pitted dates.

It sounds like a lot of work, but it only takes a few minutes. You now have fresh almond milk to add to your smoothies. I keep the left over nut meal and make raw cookies in my food dehydrator.

Sweet Potato Bites

- 4 sweet potatoes
- 2 tbsp. cinnamon
- 2 tbsp. turmeric
- 2 tbsp. curry powder
- ¼ cup virgin coconut oil

Cube the sweet potatoes into small square chunks, and then toss in the cinnamon, curry powder, turmeric, and coconut oil. Coat all the sweet potatoes with the sauce, and place them into the oven preheated to 450 degrees for about 1.5 hours. Let them cool and place about ten in little bags to toss into lunches in the morning. When I crave something sweet, I grab these sweet potato bites. My sweet tooth is sated.

The added benefit of snacking on sweet potatoes is they are extremely high in vitamin A, which is very important when combating acne (think Accutane and Retin-A). They also have a tremendous amount of fiber for optimal digestive health, so a person naturally feels fuller without consuming a high amount of calories.

For protein, I generally eat chicken or fish. I cook about 5-7 pieces of chicken every few days, and steam some vegetables for late afternoon and evening meals. Vegetarians can substitute with organic soaked and sprouted legumes (Ann Wigmore wrote the classic book on sprouting), or hemp seeds. Sprouted legumes are packed with protein and have an abundance of phytonutrients. Hemp seeds are one of nature's most perfect foods. Three tablespoons of hemp seeds will give you 11 grams of protein. Hemp seeds are also a great anti-inflammatory in that they have a 3:1 ratio of omega-6 to omega-3 fatty acids. The omega-6 fatty acid in hemp seeds is gamma linolenic acid (GLA), which is a direct building block the body utilizes to produced anti-inflammatory hormones. Hemp seeds are also noted to support a healthy metabolism and aid in weight reduction.

I work out and run a lot and find I do not feel satisfied on a vegetarian diet. I have met very active people who seem to thrive on vegan or vegetarian diets, but I have tried several times and feel I am not at my optimum health when protein is purely from plant sources.

Additionally, I do not eat legumes; they are hard on my digestive system. It has been theorized that legumes have similar effects on the digestive system as grains. That is, they have proteins that may irritate to the gut as well as protease inhibitors and anti-nutrients. When your digestive system has these types of reactions, it can cause inflammation in the system, which, in turn, can exacerbate acne symptoms.

I also mix different fruits and vegetables into my smoothies and meals. If I am really craving some variety, I select foods from the aforementioned alkaline list and mix them into my meals as well. Even when I do switch it up, I prefer to keep my meals simple with minimal prep time. Simplicity negates any excuse not to eat clean throughout the week.

So, there you have it—my clean and acne-free diet plan. I am not going to lie; initially, the diet switch may result in a few headaches and craving for sweets will ensue. However, with a little dedication, such carbohydrate cravings will diminish and your skin will start to glow. Also, simple meal plans such as these still allow time in the morning to perfect yourself into the goddess of a diva you are. Now, who does not love the idea of that!

Chapter 7

Super Foods for the Thriving Diva

To add extra nutrition to my diet, I incorporate super foods into my smoothies to give them well . . . super powers! My favorite super power booster is maca root. Maca root has literally changed my life. How can a funny named root change someone's life?

Maca is a root vegetable grown in the high Andes of Bolivia and Peru. It is an adaptogenic herb, which means it works with the body's natural rhythms to help with rebuilding weak immune systems, re-mineralizing poorly nourished bodies, and increasing energy and endurance.

More specifically, Maca is an endocrine adaptogenic. The endocrine system is a collection of glands that produce chemical messengers called hormones, which are essential for normal bodily functions. Maca can support endocrine health by helping the body produce and regulate vital hormones for optimal health and well-being.

In today's world—where most of us are stressed, sleep deprived, and undernourished—our hormones can become unbalanced. When our hormones are imbalanced, problems such as acne, depression, and irregular menses can affect the quality of our lives. I am a first-hand witness to this fact.

When I would experience premenstrual syndrome (PMS) prior to maca, I would actually become a completely different person. Feeling completely emotional and out-of-control, every little thing that would be no big deal any other time of the month would send me into a tailspin.

I can remember sitting in the parking lot of my gym, sending about twenty insane text messages to the man I am in-love with. He commented, "He was happy to see I could entertain myself with a one-way correspondence." Not the best way to keep a guy around.

I experienced this vicious cycle for nearly four years. I gave birth to two babies back-to-back, went through a divorce, self-employed, and was completely emotionally taxed and sleep-deprived. I was on an emotional hormonal rollercoaster that left me feeling depressed, isolated, and emotionally-overloaded.

I awakened one day, looked into the mirror, completely unhappy and exhausted. I knew I could not keep living this way. I felt I was living an altered life and no longer wanted to be the girl playing the starring role. From that moment, I made a pact with myself to get better. So, I bought every book on hormonal health I could find, and surfed blogs about herbs and homeopathic methods for treating hormonal imbalances.

One night, while surfing the web, I came across maca root. I started reading testimonials from women who were just like me. They claimed they started taking maca and clouds of depression and emotional unease starting lifting from them.

For me, about three weeks into taking maca root, I started to feel like a completely different person. I slept better and started feeling more optimistic about life. Best of all, I stopped having erratic emotional mood swings; I could not believe it! I felt happy and optimistic for the first time in years.

On top of the advantages of feeling rejuvenated and optimistic, my skin no longer developed large cysts around the jaw area during my menstrual cycle. Maca root is still a mainstay in my diet; it has become an emotional security blanket. I travel with it, carry a bottle of it in my purse, and if I have to check my luggage when flying, I pour some in a plastic baggie and take it on the plane with me.

I know it is a little obsessive, but I was the girl, who sent over twenty text messages to a very hot guy from my gym parking lot. Do some research on maca root as well. It appears maca root not only helps bring back an emotional hemostasis to the body, it also helps relieve menopausal symptoms. It is also being used by athletes for greater stamina and endurance.

My other favorite super food is chia seeds. I look for what I call *perfect foods* with a very high nutritional value and easy diet implementation. I stumbled across the nutritional benefits of chia seeds while reading an excellent book entitled *Born To Run*, a non-fictional novel about a reporter looking for a tribe of super-runners called the Tarahumara.

The Tarahumara are legendary for having a phenomenal ability to run great distances at very fast paces. The reporter noticed the Tarahumara drank a strange-looking beverage of chia seeds mixed with lime and water.

Being the curious creature I am, I put down my book and researched chia seeds. I was very excited to discover they fall under my perfect food category. With the click of a button, I ordered three pounds online.

I tend to be a little impatient, so I called Whole Foods to see if they carried chia seeds and sure enough they did.

I added chia seeds to the arsenal of nutrients loaded into my morning smoothie.

Why are these little babies so amazing and the preferred choice of ancient warriors? The chia seed (*Salvia hispanina L*) is a gluten-free, low carbohydrate, complete protein that is loaded with vegetarian omega-3 fatty acids. This seed is also a concentrated source of macronutrients. Even when I am traveling, I carry a small bag with me and down them with a small glass of water. Also, if you want to add a delicious yet healthy snack to your diet you can make chia seed pudding.

Chia Seed Pudding

- 2 cups of fresh almond milk
- 1/3 cup of chia seeds
- 1 tsp of cinnamon
- 1 tbsp of vanilla
- 2 tbsp of maple syrup

Sometimes I throw in some raw cacao nibs.

Mix together almond milk, cinnamon, vanilla, and maple syrup, and then with a whisk slowly mix in the chia seeds. Let the chia seeds sit for 10 to15 minutes stirring occasionally. Put in the refrigerator overnight. In the morning you have a fresh batch of chia seed pudding. Chia seed pudding will last about 3 to 4 days in the refrigerator.

Another wonder food I absolutely love is bone broth. I know what you must be thinking—no, I do not put it in my smoothies. I do, however, incorporate it into almost everything else I eat. Bone broth is chalked full of minerals, such as calcium, magnesium, phosphorus, potassium, sulfate, and fluoride. The best part of bone broth is it is not synthetically derived, so our bodies can readily assimilate the minerals in the broth.

To make bone broth, go to your local health food store or butcher and asked for femur bones. I usually buy about four pounds. I put the femur bones in a crock pot and cover with filtered water and about one-half cup of apple cider vinegar. Adding apple cider vinegar is important because the acid pulls all the yummy minerals out of the bones.

I let the bones simmer for nearly 24 hours before straining them, then add more water to the crock pot. I keep doing this until the bones have dissolved. There is always a pot of bones brewing on my countertop.

One batch of four-pound bones usually lasts ten days or so. I usually keep straining the broth out to make soups or add to my vegetable stir fry mixes, and then add more water to fill the pot back up. On days when I am feeling more depleted than others, I drink the broth like I would tea. It tastes a little odd, but I feel great afterwards and usually sleep really well because my system is relaxed by all the minerals.

Bone broth is not only good for re-mineralizing systems suffering with acne; it also has anti-aging benefits as well. Bone broth can be a fabulous part of an anti-aging diet due to the ligaments, tendon, marrow, and skin bursting with collagen. Our collagen levels decline with age and we usually start seeing a loss of suppleness in the skin; declining levels of collagen influence a decline in connective tissue.

With high amounts of collagen in our system, we can give our bodies the tools needed to help restore our connective tissue; thus, replenishing a vibrant suppleness to the skin. In order for bone broth to really be collagen rich, add chicken feet, joints, and knuckles for added super powers—it sounds like a witch's brew, but your skin will be reap the magical rewards.

Here is a quick soup recipe I love to make with my bone broth. It literally takes me five minutes.

Tomato Basil Soup

- 4 cups of bone broth
- 1 cup of fresh basil
- 2 cans of organic tomato sauce
- 1 can of organic tomato paste

I mix all these ingredients into my blender and add pepper. I store the soup in a large glass container in my refrigerator. Each morning, I heat some up and put it in a thermos to drink after my smoothies.

This soup is loaded with the super antioxidant lycopene, which fights inflammation as well as is acclaimed as an anti-cancer agent. Lycopene is released when tomatoes are cooked, so my tomato basil soup is not only chalked full of minerals from the delicious bone broth, but it is also brimming with bountiful amounts of lycopene.

Another way to incorporate bone broth into diet is to add it to protein and vegetable dishes. The following is a common dish I will incorporate into my weekly meal plans.

Bone Broth Delight

- 4 ounces of chicken
- ½ sweet potato

- 1 cup of steamed vegetables
- 2 cups of bone broth

I mix this all up in a bisphenol A-free (BPA) container and heat it for lunch or dinner. Be creative and add as many different types of herbs and spices as you would like.

Last, I cannot leave a chapter about super powers without mentioning the anti-inflammatory super hero cayenne pepper *(capsicum).* Cayenne pepper is the circulatory system's best friend. This super pepper can kick metabolism into fat-burning overdrive.

Cayenne pepper can help achieve this super status by boosting metabolism and increasing blood flow. Cayenne pepper can also aid in the elimination of toxic build up from the system, which, in turn, has a detoxifying effect on the body as a whole. Everyday I'm always researching and learning about new super foods to incorporate into my diet to help fight acne and other inflammatory conditions. You can stay up to date with my latest findings at: skinlogic.us/blog/.

Chapter 8

What About Travel?

I am frequently asked by clients in my acne clinic how to maintain a healthy diet while traveling. This can be tricky, but with the right preparation, it is attainable. I generally make some protein bars to take with me on the plane.

Here is a great recipe I created to get me through many long flights without having to eat airplane food.

Dawn's Super Granola Bars

- 3 whole eggs
- 2 cups of gluten free oatmeal
- ½ cup of almond butter
- ½ cup of hemp powder
- ½ cup of chia seeds
- ¼ cup of coconut oil
- 2 mashed bananas
- 2 tbsp. of vanilla extract
- 1 tbsp. of cinnamon
- Some organic dark chocolate (if your skin likes you afterwards)

Preheat the oven to 375 degrees. While the oven is heating up, mix all the ingredients together. Mix the wet ingredients in first, and then add the dry. Then spread the mixture onto a baking sheet lined with parchment paper. Let the mixture cook for about thirty-five minutes, and then take them out of the oven and let them cool.

Raw Version

You can make the granola bars raw by omitting the egg and adding a ½ cup of flax seed to bind the ingredients. Soak the flax seeds in water for an hour or until the liquid is absorbed, then add the flax seeds to the rest of the ingredients.

The other modification is instead of cooking the granola bars you will put them in a food dehydrator at 110 degrees for 6 to 8 hours. You can also make the granola bars into ½ inch balls and make cookies. For cookies you will want to dehydrate for 12 to 14 hours.

This generally makes enough bars to last one week. Cut them into squares and store them in the refrigerator. Each morning or when traveling, I grab a few bars and throw them into my purse. We now have a healthy, filling snack to get us through our long (or short) flights—oh, make sure to drinks a lot of water during your flight.

Another great way to ensure looking fabulous when getting off a flight is to pack a quart of coconut water in your luggage (if you check it). Consume a quart of coconut water after your flight to rehydrate your system; I have found I feel less jet-lagged.

So, what do we do when we land? Find the nearest Jamba Juice or something equivalent. Get a large carrot juice and oatmeal to tide you over until you are settled. Also, download applications onto a cellular telephone to find healthy restaurants. Most restaurants will accommodate your requests.

When eating out, I stick to salads, vegetables, and lean protein. I have never had a problem with the chef taking off some fancy sauce to prepare a piece of lean meat with steamed vegetables. I also opt for a large salad with vinegar and oil, and a protein dish of fish or lean meat.

When I am really in a pinch, I will get the protein plate at a Starbucks. I have been known to grab five protein plates, and toss them into my purse (I pay of course); especially, if I know I am going to be on the go.

Also, pop into a local grocery store to pick up some nuts, fresh fruit, and avocados to get some healthy fat into your diet. I also recently purchased a travel blender. I will grab some fresh fruit from the breakfast bar at the hotel where I am staying, and then go to my room to blend it with juice and protein powder.

Protein powders are also a necessity when traveling. I pack bags of whey protein powder, hemp protein powder, and packets of dried super greens such as spirulina and chlorella. I can add these ingredients into the smoothie I make to ensure I am taking in all my nutrients and antioxidants for the day. This leads to my next obsession—supplements.

CHAPTER 9

Supplements, Supplements, Supplements

"The doctor of the future will give no medicine, but will interest her or his patients in the care of the human frame, in a proper diet, and the cause and prevention of disease."

—*Thomas A. Edison*

I have a love affair with herbs and supplements. I have been consuming knowledge from books about herbs and supplements since I can remember. When I was a student at the University of California, Berkeley (UC Berkeley), I spent my free time at the local herb and supplement shops asking questions until the salesperson or herbalist on duty would ignore me or pretend to have other pressing things to attend to, which they probably did.

My fascination still continues to this day. A friend always makes fun of me, joking that my suitcase has more supplements and skin care products than clothing.

She jokes, "How are you ever going to get a boyfriend with a suitcase that looks like that? People are going to think you're an eccentric nut."

"Well, I totally own my eccentric nuttiness," I reply. "I just have to find a man who is as passionate about supplements and skin care as I am."

Seriously, there is some amazing new research going on in this field that is completely changing the way scientists and doctors are looking at aging, degenerative diseases, as well as inflammatory diseases and skin issues.

This field is called the science of nutrigenomics. Scientists are researching how the right kinds of supplementation and herbs can actually change our gene expression. Author, Dr. Perricone, has done a lot of research in this area; I highly recommend reading some of his latest research to learn more about how doctors and scientists are discovering the right foods and supplementation can reverse a lot of inflammatory conditions within the body.

What the heck does this have to do with acne? Well, acne is an inflammatory disease, and all the nutrients that change gene expression also reduce inflammation in the body. The added benefit is while we are fighting acne, we can also slow down the aging process and perhaps side-step some manifesting illnesses. My must-have supplements are as follows:

- A Food-based Multi-Vitamin
- Fish oil
- Astaxanthin
- Éminence VitaSkin Vitamins, Clear Skin
- Éminence VitaSkin Vitamins, Firm Skin
- Éminence VitaSkin Vitamins, Clam Skin

Why do I choose these as my must-have heavy-hitters? Well, I love food-based multi-vitamins because they have an advantage over their synthetic counterparts. Our body recognizes foods; therefore, can more easily assimilate the nutrients into our system.

I have also found most food-based organic supplement companies stay current with the latest research and constantly update their formulas to provide consumers the best multi-vitamin for optimal health. Further, most companies that promote and sell organic goods generally strive for the highest organic and sustainable farming practices and have fair trade practices with farmers and workers, who they employ and do business with around the world.

Fish oil is a must-have for anyone trying to combat inflammation in the system. When I am under a tremendous amount of stress and traveling a lot, I double my fish oil intake. In our modern diet, we consume high amounts of processed foods—dairy and meat—which make our diet high in Omega-6 fatty acid and low in Omega-3 fatty acids.

High levels of Omega-6 fatty acid can be a contributing component to high levels of inflammation in the system. Since most of us do not consume enough foods high in Omega-3 fatty acids, such as flax, chia seeds, and salmon, it becomes imperative to consume fish oils as well as other rich sources of Omega-3 fatty acids to control inflammation in the system.

Once we start consuming high levels of Omega-3 fatty acids, our skin will appear to have more suppleness, acne lesions may start decreasing, and we experience an overall calming of inflammation in the skin. Some clients have also noted when they started taking high levels of Omega-3 fatty acids, they noticed their skin appeared firmer and cheekbones seemed higher.

Astaxanthin has been getting a lot of press lately. It is quickly becoming the next super star in the world of supplementation. Dr. Mehmet Oz even did a segment on *The Dr. Oz Show* about the positive effects of astaxanthin.

Why is this supplement so amazing? Astaxanthin is a carotenoid that is abundant in single-cell microalga. When consumed by shrimp and salmon species, astaxanthin stores in their bodies and gives them the rich orange and pink hues we associate with them.

Astaxanthin is currently being touted as the most powerful antioxidant currently known and studied by man. It is considered to be one thousand times more powerful than vitamin E in combating free radial damage in the body and on the skin. Free radical damage occurs when an oxygen goes crazy and loses an electron (like me when I experience PMS), and it creates a singlet oxygen, which ages us and causes inflammation in the body. This is really bad. Who wants wrinkles, inflammation, and acne—a girl's worst nightmare!

Astaxanthin can negate the crazies and mitigate the damage of reactive oxygen species (ROS) or free radicals, which—in the game of aging and inflammation—makes us very happy. Therefore, by blocking the negative effects of ROS we can combat acne and aging, this can be a key component to overall skin and physical health. There are some studies floating around on the internet that claim astaxanthin can also reduce pigmentation and wrinkles, as well as restore firmness to the skin and create natural ultraviolet (UV) protection.

Another supplement for acne is Clear Skin VitaSkin Vitamins, by Éminence Organic Skin Care. I take these vitamins along with Mag07, a colon cleanser, before I go to bed each night. Clear skin vitamins are probiotic-based supplements that also contain zinc, borage seed oil, and *NutraFlora®*.

Probiotics are becoming the next super hero in the war against acne. Probiotics are healthy bacteria, which propagate in the bowels; however, in today's world where most of us take too many antibiotics for acne and other conditions, our healthy intestinal flora decreases. When this occurs, a host of other problems ensue.

When healthy bacteria levels have been compromised, digestive problems and constipation result. When our bodies are constipated, toxins build up in the system, which leads to our bodies eliminating toxins through the skin and exacerbating acne symptoms.

By restoring healthy bacteria to the bowels by adding probiotics to our diet, we can more efficiently eliminate toxins from our system, which can help manage elevating acne symptoms. Éminence Clear Skin vitamins are my preference because they do not have to be refrigerated—a common trait of high quality probiotics—and they have a unique pill-in-pill concept. This approach ensures its ingredients pass though the stomach, reaching the intestine for optimum absorption.

I take my probiotics along with Mag 07. Mag 07 is a powerful colon cleanser, which creates a very rich oxygenated environment, and in turn, makes the probiotics more effective. Healthy bacteria thrive in a rich, oxygenated environment. Most diseases resulting from unhealthy bacteria thrive in an anaerobic (non-oxygenated) environment.

By creating an aerobic environment, we reap the highest benefits of a probiotic supplement. There arc many high quality Mag 07 supplements available online or in local health food stores. I highly recommend this combination before bed for optimal well-being; I take it one-half hour before I go to bed with water.

Also a proven mineral to help clear up acne, zinc helps support the immune system and calm inflammation in the body. The other amazing ingredient in this supplement is borage seed oil, which helps dilute sebum production. It is also very high in gamma-linolenic acid (GLA). Shown to improve skin conditions, GLA also helps heal eczema and psoriasis duc to its anti-inflammatory properties.

I also take the Firm and Calm Skin vitamins, by Éminence Organic Skin Care because what girl is not concerned with aging? The standouts in Firm Skin vitamins are sea buckthorn and vitamin A. I take sea buckthorn internally as well as apply it topically.

Sea buckthorn is a beautiful, vibrant fruit grown in Canada, Asia, and parts of Europe. It is getting a lot of attention as the next big super food. What is so amazing about sea buckthorn?

Sea buckthorn is powerful at combating inflammation and toxicity in the body—two conditions that lead to aging and acne. It is high in vitamins C and E, and contains palmitoleic acid, which is a natural occurring fatty acid found in skin. Palmitoleic acid can be depleted by chronic skin conditions, aging, and acne.

Vitamin A has been well-researched as an essential nutrient for many years, and has been well-documented as an immune boosting nutrient that guards against viral, bacterial, and parasitic overgrowth in our systems. I could fill an entire book with the advantages of vitamin A, highlighting its key role in boosting our health to ward off diseases and aging.

I also believe in conjunction with taking vitamin A in supplement form, we should also consume as many foods as possible with high levels of vitamin A such as foods with deep orange hues, which is indicative of high beta carotene content (vitamin A).

The standouts in Calm Skin vitamins are milk thistle, green tea extract, and pine bark extract. Milk thistle is a well-known liver tonic. *Silymarin* is the power player in milk thistle, which is an antioxidant and anti-inflammatory. Recognize a trend here?

By ingesting milk thistle, we can increase our liver function and, therefore, help assist the elimination of toxic buildup. With decreased toxicity in our system, our liver can function at a more optimal level, leading to an overall healthier functioning immune system.

We have all read numerous articles about the amazing powers of green tea, which has the super antioxidants cathecins; particularly, one of the major cathecins: epigallocatechin-3-gallate (EGCG). These agents have been researched and are believed to help fight cancer cells by not allowing them to enter the body.

Other benefits of green tea, touted in the press, are its thermogenic effects on the body. These effects are said to increase metabolism, aid in weight loss, as well as support the immune system and fight free radicals. It may be safe to say, we should not only protect our cells by taking green tea in our supplements, but we should also replace our coffee with copious amounts of green tea throughout the day.

Pine bark extract, also known as pycnogenol, is derived from the maritime pine tree (*pinus pinaster*). It contains a chemical called proanthocyanidins, which is said to be a powerful antioxidant that fights inflammation and blocks the action of free radial damage in the body.

According to a study conducted by the Leibniz Research Institute for Environmental Medicine, in Dusseldorf, Germany, where twenty women, ages 55-60, were given seventy-five milligrams of pine bark a day for twelve weeks. These women experienced a 44 percent increase in hyaluronic acid, 25 percent increases in elasticity, and 6 percent improvement in the smoothness of their skin. These outcomes were pretty amazing.

So, there you have it; all the key nutrients beneficial to help calm inflammation in the body, thus, reducing the amount of acne lesions on the skin. I have seen some of my clients change their whole diet and supplementation program, only to have the worst break of their lives. This reprieve is only temporary though.

The skin, the largest organ of the body, is one of the vehicles the body uses to purge toxins. Keeping this in mind, it only seems natural after years of toxic sludge built up; our bodies need to eliminate it before achieving optimum health. If patient, within a few weeks our skin will start to calm down and have a newfound glow to it.

Trust me, I know from my own experience; going through this initial phase can be very stressful. However, making the suggested lifestyle changes outlined will have tremendous long-term benefits on your health, confidence, and overall well-being.

CHAPTER 10

Colonics . . . Skin Brushing . . . Exercise . . . Oh, My!

"All disease begins in the gut"

—Hippocrates

After embarking on this clean eating and supplementation program, we need to think about further cleansing the years of toxin build up accumulated in our digestive tract with colonics. What the heck is colonics?

Colonic hydrotherapy is administered when a trained colonic hydro therapist inserts a tube in the rectum, filling the colon and abdomen with warm water. The water is then released along with any toxic build up accumulated within the digestive system. Yes, it may sound strange, but while seeing substances purge from your body, you will become a believer.

When I attended my first session, I thought I was going to be a superior client with an exemplary colon that purged nothing. Heck, I eat a fifty percent raw food diet; I do not drink alcohol, eat sugar, and, hell, I do not even drink coffee. Boy was I wrong! There were all kinds of toxic waste purging from my body!

Before the start of my first session, the hydro therapist explained a toxic liver will excrete yellowish bile and a toxic gallbladder will excrete greenish bile. Therefore, I would become aware of what was coming out of my body as it passed through a clear tube during the release phase.

I was so shocked during my second fill and release; my body was excreting deep yellowish bile. The therapist explained I had a lot of toxic build up in my liver. She said no matter how healthy we are we live in a toxic environment. What is stuck in our digestive tract and liver comes from years of accumulated toxins caused by diet, stress, and other environmental factors.

After my first session, I felt really great and signed up for another visit. The colon hydro therapist explained it takes nearly ten sessions to rid the body of all toxic sludge. Most people come back every quarter for maintenance.

I highly recommend this treatment, especially if a colon hydro therapist is accessible. It is another level of detoxification to ensure our bodies are functioning optimally. Additionally, I highly recommend after each session to get a massage to further relax and de-stress the body.

Skin brushing is also an important part of our daily detoxification program; a skin brush can be bought at most health food stores. I recommend skin brushing for a few minutes in the evening before getting into the bathtub or shower.

When using a skin brush, make long, circular strokes on the arms, legs, and back while working inwards toward the heart. If we are really brave, we can do hot-cold therapy to accelerate circulation and blood flow through the body.

Simply run the water in the shower hot then cold for a few minutes. Asides from removing dead skin cells and increasing blood flow, skin brushing also stimulates the lymph and hormonal system. This activity can be beneficial for our overall health.

I am also a proponent of bio-magnetic therapy. We have all been taught the earth is surrounded by a magnetic field. Scientists have discovered the earth's magnetic field has been decreasing in recent years, which means a decrease in our bodies receiving sufficient magnetic energy.

Why is this important? Magnetic therapy is recognized by many scientists as having therapeutic healing properties to keep the body in balance. As we know, chronic conditions such as acne can arise when our bodies are out of balance.

When magnetic therapy brings our body back into balance, it is believed to help maintain increased oxygen levels, increased blood flow, and restoration of the body's pH balance. When I started to sleep on magnets, I had more restful sleep as well as felt more energized each morning.

I also magnetize my beverages with a magnet pad. By magnetizing beverages, it is said to raise their pH balance and, subsequently, restore a proper pH balance to the body.

Remember, an overly acidic body can lead to inflammation and chronic acne conditions. Learn more about magnetic therapy at www.MagneticServices.com.

Lastly, exercise is one of the most important contributors to overall health. Believe me, when I have had a long day the last thing I feel like doing is working out. However, I still head to the gym or track. Plus, there has never been a time when I finish my workout and did not feel better than when I started it.

My workouts are probably a little more hard core than most. I have been known to run marathons and ultra-marathons. I am not asking you to run a 50km race, but getting at least thirty minutes of exercise a day will help make your life a sunnier place to reside.

The upside is having a fabulous derriere to flaunt in the summer time. What diva does not want to look fabulous in a sexy bikini?

The major benefit of exercise, aside from a beautiful backside, is it is the most effective way to continuously rid the body of toxins. When we exercise we increase circulation of blood flow, lymph, and we sweat. When we workout more strenuously, we breathe deeply, which relaxes the body and mind to release endorphins—happy hormones.

There are different types of workout programs in the world. I like variation, so I mix it up; I run, do yoga, take a dance class, lift weights, and spin, to name a few. Keep exercise interesting and fun, so you are more likely to stick with it. Who wants to go to the gym day in and day out, toiling away at the same routine?

I also recommend working out with a goal. Try training for a 10k, then perhaps a one-half marathon, then a full marathon, which leads up to 26.2 miles of blissful running. Sign up and compete in a bikini contest. I competed in a National Physique Committee International Federation of BodyBuilders (NPC IBFF) Bikini Competition. It was one of the most empowering and challenging athletic endeavors of my life.

I trained for a whole year, changing my diet and lifting heavy weights like a mad woman to feel confident competing on stage. It was such an amazing experience to get on stage after all the hard work and compete against a group of breathtakingly beautiful athletic women.

So, make working out fun. Life is supposed to be fun. Live a healthy clean lifestyle and have a blast doing it—just be creative! Instead of heading out to the local eatery and regretting the burger and curly fries when you step on the scale, opt for inviting friends over to cook a healthy and interesting online recipe. Drink fresh apple, carrot, or ginger juice in wine glasses. Celebrate and spread the word of health wherever you go.

You may initially be the odd bird in the bunch, but friends will start to see your newfound confidence and join you. Being different will spark the curiosity of others. I travel with my food and a gym bag pretty much wherever I go. People are always curious and ask what is in my containers. Sometimes people laugh, but most think it inspiring.

I remember once when I was standing in the taxi line at the Las Vegas airport, a group of guys asked what was in my cooler.

I laughed and said, "Sweet potatoes, carrot juice, and chicken."

One of the guys said, "Seriously?"

"Yes," I replied, "seriously."

I then added, "I might be the only girl in Las Vegas who will not drink, gamble, or have sex."

He was so taken by my confidence to live life by my own rules with no embarrassment; he looked me up on Facebook to ask me out. I did not go out with him, but he complimented me saying, "I was one of the most beautiful, bubbly, confident women he had ever met."

I do not know about you, but I will take that kind of compliment any day! Being confident in your body and health translates in every other area of your life, no matter what you are doing, no matter where you are.

Chapter 11

Extra Detox Ideas for the Eccentric-Minded

This next concept may seem a little over the top for some. Even my oldest son calls this my "space suit unit," and then proceeds to tell me I am not like the other mommies. I am still not quite sure whether this is a compliment or not.

What is he referring to when he describes my space suit unit? He is talking about my *FAR infrared thermal energy heat sauna blanket*. FAR infrared energy is credited with helping the body rid itself of heavy metals and toxins, aid in weight loss, promote cellulite reduction, ease insomnia symptoms, and reduce the negative effects of stress.

I decided to purchase a FAR infrared blanket to aide in stress reduction and insomnia, which I have struggled with for as long as I can remember. When my insomnia gets really bad, my skin and health suffer.

I have never wanted to take sleep aids, since I have been struggling with sleep issues for several years. I also did not want to become dependent on something I felt would negatively impact my health.

I have tried every homeopathic remedy for insomnia on the market, yet nothing has helped. After doing research on FAR infrared, I figured I would give it a try. I was so excited when I received it in the mail.

The blanket looked a bit strange; I was a little nervous the first time I used it. However, after approximately fifteen minutes in my space suit unit, I started to relax and sweat—boy, do you sweat!

I can see why they say it may help with detoxification and weight loss. Presumably, I sweat out half my body weight in my first thirty-minute session. Okay, maybe I did not sweat out half my body weight, but I sweat out at least a pound.

After about a week of lying in my FAR infrared blanket every night, I started to sleep better. I do not know if it has a placebo effect, but I am sticking with it. Plus, after thirty minutes of sweating profusely, I feel great.

I am totally addicted to this thing. I might even have to buy an extra suitcase for my space suit unit, so I can have it with me even when I travel. Although, I may get strange looks when going through US Customs. I will simply shrug my shoulders and say, "It's my security blanket." I think with all the other strange things floating around in my luggage, they may just think I am a really strange girl.

Well, if my readers ever have a long layover at the airport, and happen to see me, just say, "Hi." I will let you detox with me in the lounge as we nosh on super chia granola bars.

To go one step further, do not only detox your body, but also detox your nervous system. To detox your nervous system, I highly recommend finding a chiropractor who practices Network Spinal Analysis (NSA). You may already think I am way nutty at this point, but hear me out.

Network Spinal Analysis is a type of chiropractic care that focuses on touching the spine in non-invasive ways. It helps the body create energy pathways, so the nervous system can better process and release stressors that lead to an unbalanced physical state.

I had the pleasure of interviewing Dr. Bryce Renshaw, who practices a form of this type of chiropractic care, to ask him to break this approach down into digestible consideration. He explained many of us walk around with a constant stream of low level mental chatter. He described how this low level mental chatter takes over our physical energy fields and starts directing our lives to create stress patterns that can manifest into physical and emotional imbalance.

This state distresses the whole system because "eternally your emotional environment is screaming for security and stabilization." Dr. Renshaw further explained, "Network Spinal Analysis helps rebuild the house you thought was safe that you built for yourself as a child from age two to where you are now."

This emotional house we have built for ourselves was created on the foundation given to us as children by the emotional patterning demonstrated by our parents or caregivers. Unfortunate for some of us, the building blocks of our emotional centers have their foundation centered in patterns created while witnessing dysfunctional dynamics between primary caregivers and their environment.

Network Spinal Analysis helps to create a healthier dynamic within the body as a whole by using the breath wave, which NSA is based upon. By creating these breath waves, we create a space to re-pattern ourselves energetically, so we can re-create a healthier foundation to lead a more energetically open life.

When we feel more energetically open, we feel more balanced mentally and physically. This is due to the fact that the spinal cord is an extension of the brain; everything in our environment—external and internal—is interconnected with our nervous system.

How does all this tie in with acne? Well, my acne symptoms were not only a symptom of the high levels of cellular inflammation within my body, but they were also linked to high levels of emotional stress, which causes high levels of cortisol. In turn, high levels of cortisol cause hormonal imbalances that can lead to acne related symptoms.

Network Spinal Analysis gave me tools to deal with the emotional stressors of daily life. I also have tools to deal with residual emotional patterning from my childhood; thus, balancing me out as a whole.

Chapter 12

The First Commandment—Love Thy Aesthetician!

I am an aesthetician and I believe I have the greatest job on the planet; I may be a little partial, but seriously, a great aesthetician can really transform a person's skin. I have had several clients, who have walked in my clinic with some of the worst cases of cystic acne and low self-confidence. However, within months, I have witnessed their skin and lives transformed.

For me, there is really no better feeling in the world than when I help someone achieve the complexion he or she has always wanted. At the end of the day, my clients are more than simply clients. They are individuals, who have invited me to witness part of their journey called life.

I have seen my clients have babies and go through divorces. I have listened to many tales of travels and romantic adventures from all corners of the world. My clients have offered me opportunities and friendships that have changed me in ways I could never put into words.

Most importantly, they trusted me to help them and be part of the healing process on their clear skin journey. Wow, I *do* have a pretty amazing job!

What is the magic, which transpires for my clients between the first appointment and when they walk through the door smiling with clear, glowing skin? Well . . . a whole lot! As you can see, I do not take a traditional approach. Initially, I coach them on diet and supplementation, and then we tackle skin care.

If a client walks in with severe cystic acne, I inquire about his or her diet and stress levels. I suggest the dietary and lifestyle changes I have written about. Then I put him or her on a skin care and treatment program to fit his or her lifestyle.

The primary skin care line I stand behind is Éminence Handmade Organic Skin Care Of Hungry. I love this skin care system because it has one of the highest organic standards in the industry. Additionally, it is one of the first skin care lines in the world to have a certified Biodynamic® line.

Demeter, the only global certifying body of Biodynamic®, has certified Éminence as having the highest purity level in the skin care industry. It is fair to say, Éminence Organic Skin Care is committed to the highest organic standards in skin care.

Éminence produces pure, fresh, botanical skin care, using the freshest organic fruits, herbs, and pulps to bring outstanding results. This skin care line accomplishes this without testing on animals, using harsh chemicals, or adding parabens or sulfates to their products.

What does Biodynamic® mean? Biodynamic® Farming (*meaning life energy*) is a philosophy of farming founded by the late anthroposophist, Rudolf Steiner, in 1922 as a reaction to the heavy pesticide use and degradation of farm soil in Europe.

Steiner proposed farms be treated as closed and holistic ecosystems where all components of that system are treated as interdependent parts. Meaning, recycling plant nutrients and other nutrient sources within the farm to nourish the soil, while refraining from using any form of chemicals that would harm anything within this closed ecosystem.

I had the pleasure of sitting down to speak with Lisbeth Boger who is the Northern California representative of Éminence Organic Skin Care to talk with her about the Éminence line, its principles, and the benefits of organic and Biodynamic® farming in skin care. She explained when Éminence was brought to North America, the intention of the founder, Boldijarre Koronczay, was to bring a natural plant-based Hungarian line as opposed to an organic line.

Koronczay, a third generation master aesthetician, became passionate about natural plant-based therapies due to his struggle with leukemia as small child. His family treated his leukemia with natural and alternative medicine. So, from a young age, Koronczay became aware of the power of healing the body and skin through plant-based ingredients and therapies. However, when bringing a natural plant-based line to North America, Koronczay did not realize Hungarian farming practices, as opposed to North American ones, were what we considered organic.

Hungary was behind the iron curtain and very poor during the time America experienced its industrial revolution. While the American farming industry was being industrialized, the farming industry in Hungary was too poor to have access to advanced technology introduced to the farming industry in the United States during this time. Consequently, Hungarian farms were organic because their soil was not exposed to heavy pesticide uses and the modern industrial methods of crop growth.

Because of this, the nutrient content of the Hungarian soil was not depleted by heavy pesticide use. In conjunction with this, Hungary used to sit beneath the ocean, so her soil content is very nutritionally dense. According to Boger, "The soil in Hungry is so rich and so black it's amazing."

Hungary's rich soil, coupled with its climate, yields extremely rich and nutritionally dense crops. The benefit of this for skin care is applying higher concentrations of botanicals onto the skin to help correct skin issues as well as calm inflammatory conditions caused by external stressors.

I asked Boger when choosing an organic skin care product, why she would recommend Éminence Organic Skin Care over other organic skin care brands. She told me we need to think about the crops used in the Éminence line just as we would think about growing grapes to make wine.

Wine can only be grown in certain regions in the world to maintain the quality and depth we associate with a high quality glass of wine, the same goes for skin care. Boger stated, "Éminence is a Terrier of organic skin care."

If Éminence tried to grow crops anywhere else in the world, they would not get the same concentration of nutrients. Éminence farms even superseded their traditional farming practices when they created their Biodynamic® line, which is 20 percent more nutritionally dense than their traditional organic line.

The Biodynamic® plant having 20 percent more nutrition than an organic plant gives a person, who is struggling with sensitivity and inflammatory problems, the purest, most concentrated ingredients to feed his or her skin. These Biodynamic® crops, Boger explains, "Are sprayed with high concentrations of vitamin C and inter-planted with other plants to keep bugs off. They are even planted at different root depths every year to draw different nutrition from the soil. These methods yield such a hearty and nutritionally-dense plant that even in mid-winter; they are twice the size of regular plants grown under conventional methods."

I told Boger this all sounds wonderful, but asked what is said to the person, who is struggling with acne issues and he or she is made to believe he or she needs to put harsh chemicals on his or her skin in order to get relief from symptoms? How is a plant going to have a small enough molecular structure to drive down into the skin as effectively as other traditional chemicals known to have a smaller molecular structure, hence, appear to be more effective?

She advised me I had posed a good question and "Éminence exposes everything to ultrasound, which breaks down the molecules into smaller pieces so you get better product penetration, which is more readily absorbed into the skin."

By using plant-based products on the skin to treat conditions such as acne, you may not get as fast a result as you would with traditional methods such as benzoyl peroxide and chemically-based therapies, but in the long-run, by using plant-based ingredients, you help to rebuild a healthier cell. By doing this, skin is brought back into balance. The long-term benefits of putting the skin back into balance are: less inflammation, less oil, more hydration, and an overall healthy, dewy appearance.

What are the standout ingredients in these products that are beneficial for the acne suffer? Although I know it is a mainstay ingredient in the fight against acne, I generally never put any of my clients on benzoyl peroxide because it is very harsh on the skin and causes excessive dryness and skin sensitivity.

I will use benzoyl peroxide as a last resort, but try hard to refrain from adding it to any client's skin care regime. If I end up having to add it to a client's homecare program, I try to only have them on it for a few months. Eventually, I switch the person over to products that contain willow bark and tree tea oil, which I prefer as my antibacterial fighting agent.

The other reason I try to avoid benzoyl peroxide and using other harsh ingredients for long periods of time is when acne is treated by bombarding the skin repeatedly with harsh chemicals, the root of the problem has not been addressed. Believing acne is an inflammatory condition and a systemic problem; I would do a disservice to my clients if I continued them on the pathway of topical skin annihilation. I would, in a sense, simply turn off the fire alarm and have them remain in a burning building. That is, I would be ignoring the deeper issues regarding why they were struggling with acne in the first place.

If I myself kept on the pathway of antibiotics and harsh topical medications, I never would have discovered I was gluten intolerant. The long-term ramification of consuming gluten when you have an allergy is disastrous. It can lead to long-term inflammation in the body, which can lead to a host of other inflammatory conditions. It may not be as fast way of achieving clear skin, but in the long-run, health benefits overall.

The other benefit of using plant-based products on acne is we are not continuing to bog down the immune system with yet another chemical cocktail. The average women puts over two hundred different chemicals on her body when applying personal care products each morning.

When a person is suffering from acne, his or her immune system is already under attack and producing high levels of inflammation. Then why continue to overload it while not addressing the issues causing acne in the first place?

The following are the key ingredients, which have helped my clients achieve clear skin:

Niacinamide, also known as vitamin B3, has been shown to have some amazing skin benefits. Recent claims have stated niacinamide may help reduce fine lines; help diminish pigmentation; and, at concentrations of 4 percent, be just as effective, if not more, than topical antibiotics without the side effects for treating acne.

The other benefit of using niacinamide over topical antibiotics is niacinamide has been shown to help retain moisture in the skin. Whereas many traditional acne ingredients strip the epidermal barrier of the skin, causing dryness and irritation.

To ensure moisturizer has a 4 percent concentration of niacinamide, I recommend ordering niacinamide powder to add to moisturizer. I order my niacinamide from Skin Actives at www.skinactives.com. It is very inexpensive; half a tube of niacinamide from Skin Actives makes a 4 percent concentration in a two fluid ounce moisturizer. I also noticed when I started using a 4 percent concentration of niacinamide, my acne scars started to diminish more rapidly.

Glycolic acid is an alpha hydroxyl acid derived from sugar cane. It is the only *alpha hydroxy acid* (AHA) that has a small enough molecular structure to penetrate through the cell walls.

The benefit of this action is when applied topically to the skin it loosens the glue that holds the cells together.

When these bonds are loosened, it causes the skin cells to turnover at a more rapid rate. The benefits of this are: it gives the skin a more even texture, it reduces the appearance of pigmentation, and it lessens the appearances of fine lines and wrinkles. Through rapid exfoliation, it also clears out the pores and helps acne reduction.

Lactic acid is another AHA derived from sour milk. It has similar benefits to glycolic, but due to its larger molecular structure, has a slower skin absorption rate, causing less irritation and dryness. This is a beneficial acid for acne suffers whose skin is too sensitive for glycolic acids.

Mandelic acid, or alpha-hydroxy benzeneacetic acid, is an AHA that has gained popularity in the past few years. Mandelic acid comes from the bitter extract of the German mandel, meaning almond. This AHA has anti-bacterial properties and helps to regulate sebum production (the film, making one's face look like an oil slick by lunchtime).

Sea buckthorn, the super berry mentioned in the supplement section, is also a wonderful topical ingredient for acne. It is loaded with over a dozen skin protecting phytosterols, carotenoids, polar lips, and Omega-7.

Sea buckthorn is said to be a powerful anti-inflammatory as well as a hormone regulator when taken orally or applied topically. Sea buckthorn also penetrates deep down into the skin, thereby, feeding the skin with a powerhouse of anti-inflammatories. Sea buckthorn also contains natural salicylic acid and is high in vitamin E, which helps break down abnormal skin growth and softens the skin.

Willow bark, or salix nigra, comes from the black willow bark tree. Willow bark is high in natural salicylic acid. Meaning, it has similar exfoliating and anti-inflammatorily properties as salicylic acids.

The anti-inflammatory properties in willow bark make it excellent for acne as well as rosacea and aging skin. Willow bark can also play a role in bringing over-exfoliated skin back into hemostasis. The bark of the willow tree protects the tree by regulating moisture content, temperature, as well as protecting it from external environmental stressors.

Azelaic acid (AA) is a hepta dicarboxylic acid derived form oleic acid in milk, fats, and potatoes. It has been shown to have an anti-bacterial effect against p. acne bacteria as well as decreasing yeast spores within the cell.

Another benefit of azelaic acid: it is has been shown to be a natural tyrosinase inhibitor. Tyrosinase is an enzyme that causes those unsightly brown spots that pop up on after an acne outbreak. Therefore, azelaic acid can be beneficial in inhibiting bacteria within the pore as well as reducing pigmentation.

Tea Tree Oil, derived from the melaleuca alternifolia plant, which is native to the Australian coast. Tea tree oil has strong anti-bacterial, antiseptic, and antifungal properties. It can be a beneficial alternative for people, who cannot tolerate the side effects common with benzoyl peroxide, such as redness, itching, and peeling.

Resorcinol is sourced from wood barks. It is a powerful agent I use on my clients with severe cystic acne. Resorcinol drives deep into the pore, producing a very strong anti-bacterial effect and, thus, is effective in calming extremely inflamed lesions. It also has skin lightening properties, so it helps reduce discoloration—a by-product of acne lesions.

On an aside note, resorcinol is an ingredient in modified Jessner peels. The line I carry for my stronger peels is Dermaquest Skin Therapy. Although Dermaquest is not an organic brand, it uses the latest scientifically-proven skin care ingredients mixed with ayurvedic (meaning the knowledge for long life) herbal wisdom to treat various skin care conditions.

Dermaquest Skin Therapy, with one of the leading chemists in the world as its founder, Sam Dhatt, is always abreast of the latest research, which allows it an advantage. Dermaquest Skin Therapy brings exceptional products to the market that contains cutting edge science while using the synergy of botanicals to deliver outstanding results.

Lastly, we have two outstanding ingredients that help rebuild the skin, plant-based retinol alternative and Swiss apple stem cells. Plant-based retinol alternative from the Anogeissus tree, resides in the lush forests of Ghana. It is believed to have the same skin benefits as retinols without the common side effects of retinols such as photosensitivity, peeling, and irritation.

How can this be? Plants that generally survive in tropical environments have to withstand very harsh and drastic climate changes.

The properties of these plants that allow them to adapt to their environment have been found to be beneficial agents to protect and slow the ageing process when applied topically to the skin. This is great news for those who are like myself and cannot tolerate retinols.

Apple stem cells, from the Swiss-grown Uttwiler Spätlauber apples, work very similar to human stem cells in maintaining and repairing the skin tissues. What is so special about the stem cells of these apples? Swiss scientists discovered the longevity of these apple stem cells long after they had fallen from their tree and shriveled up.

Studies show apple stem cells protect our cells from stress as well as well as boost our stem cell production. This is great news for the acne sufferer whose skin has been traumatized repeatedly by inflammatory acne lesions—there is hope now for baby smooth skin.

In order to visualize the difference between the previously referenced acids think of little circles linked together. The more circles linked together, the larger the molecular structure. This being said, glycolic acid has a 2-carbon chain, lactic acid has a 3-carbon chain, salicylic acid has a 6-carbon chain, and Mandelic acid has an 8-carbon chain. The larger the chain of a particular acid, the larger the molecule; the larger the molecule, the slower the absorbency rate the acid has entering into the skin.

There are many other ingredients beneficial for acneic skin, but the aforementioned I feel are the main ingredients one suffering from acne should seek out when looking for treatments and home care products. I use a combination of these ingredients in my treatment room as well as a host of other powerful antioxidants. I also incorporate technology to enhance the beneficial properties of all the ingredients I use in my treatments.

The standout products in this skin care line are as follows:

- Éminence Clear Skin Probiotic Masque
- Éminence Clear Skin Probiotic Moisturizer
- Éminence Strawberry Rhubarb Dermofoilant
- Éminence Biodynamic® Echinacea Recovery Cream
- Éminence Biodynamic® Cornflower Recovery Serum
- Éminence Bamboo Firming Fluid

CHAPTER 13

My Must-Have I Cannot Live Without Technology

I think it is very amazing that aestheticians today have the power to really transform our clients' skin. I love mixing organic ingredients with technology, having the ability to drive botanicals deep into the skin can result in mind-blowing transformations.

I have taken pictures of my clients before and after a treatment; the results are nothing less than astounding. I can lift, firm, calm and hydrate a client in sixty minutes. It is such a great feeling when a new client walks out of my treatment room completely thrilled with his or her skin transformation.

I received a lot of *wows* and *I cannot believe it!* I also get, "If you try and leave San Jose, I will hunt you down." I take this as an extreme compliment because, I always strive to bring my clients the best and most-current results-driven treatments.

How do I take a client to wow? Well, I am not going to give up my secretes of how I mix various Éminence products—you will have to come see me. Though, I will disclose the right blend of botanicals for your skin condition with the proper technology can get superb results.

The following are my top favorite pieces of equipment:

Radiancy LHE is light heat energy, using light combined with heat to treat various conditions of the skin. By combining light and heat energy, similar results can be achieved to laser resurfacing without any downtime. Using LHE in acne treatments can decrease the inflammation of acne lesions in a shorter time interval than traditional treatments without LHE.

Radiancy LHE uses a 400-430nm-wave length to create a rich oxygenated environment, which helps destroy p. acnes bacteria. Remember p. acnes bacteria feel abundantly happy in an anaerobic, or non-oxygenated, environment, so by exposing them to heat and oxygen, we can reduce the inflammation and bacteria to create a faster healing response in the acne lesion.

The following is a great treatment for those struggling with mild discoloration and moderate breakouts.

Diamond microdermabrasion uses non-surgical resurfacing techniques to help rejuvenate the skin and reduce mild acne scarring and pigmentation. The diamond tip peels the top layer of the skin, while the suction vacuums up any residual dead skin and debris.

The benefits of this action help with rejuvenation and scarring as well as reduction of pore size (we love this) and an overall glowing complexion. When diamond microdermabrasion is paired with the right treatment serums, some pretty spectacular results can be achieved.

Next is an amazing treatment to help firm the skin, clear stagnate lymphatic fluid from the face, and calm inflammation.

Cupping is a modern use of an ancient tool. Cupping therapy uses glass cups attached to a hose to create suction on the skin's surface. By gliding these cups over the surface of the skin, it causes a soft tissue release. The suction, by working deep into the soft tissue, can pull toxins and inflammation to the surface of the skin, which can then be eliminated through the lymphatic system.

The other benefits of cupping are increased blood flow to dehydrated tissues, the breakup of old scar tissue, and released congestion in old stagnant tissue. All of these benefits result in clearer, hydrated, and more youthful-looking skin.

This is by far my favorite piece of equipment; in one session I see amazing results. Clients have come in with puffiness, stagnation, and dark circles. Within one session, by draining the toxic stagnation and inflammation in the tissue, they leave with firmer, vibrant, and more defined contours in the face.

Next is a great treatment, which addresses a lot of scar tissue and active cystic lesions:

Micro derma needle roller therapy, is an amazing little torture device for acne scars. It literally resembles a medieval torture device. The derma needle is a handheld roller that has about five hundred micro needles on it, which roll over the face in segmented patterns. It is not a pleasant feeling, but the results are amazing.

I have had clients with pretty bad scarring achieve smooth, glowing skin using this little device. By creating thousands of micro-punctures in the skin, derma needle therapy promotes collagen and elastin production by wounding the skin and causing a healing response.

The other benefit of derma needling is any serums used during the derma needling session have an increased absorbency rate of up to 400 percent. This allows maximum effectiveness of any serum being used for treatments of a specific skin condition during the derma needling session.

This is a great treatment for clients who deal with scaring, but do not want the downtime caused by laser resurfacing.

How to keep skin glowing and radiant in between facial treatments:

- I recommend doing a light peel and masque once a week appropriate for your skin type.
- I highly recommend the bt-micro by Bio-Therapeutic. It is an investment, but your skin will thank you. The bt-micro allows peeling of the skin without using any harsh chemicals, and it allows for better product penetration of creams and serums.

    With continued use of the bt-micro, your skin will appear smoother, your pores will have a more refined look, and your acne lesion will start to diminish. Seriously consider having a clear skin fundraiser and buy a bt-micro. They cost around $350.

- I encourage you to wear an organic or natural mineral makeup. Now, there are so many great mineral makeup options out there that benefit the skin as well as cover up imperfections.
- Wash your makeup brushes once a week, as well as clean them with an anti-bacterial spray daily.
- Most importantly, drink lots of water. Most of us walk around in a state of dehydration. If the body is in a chronic state of dehydration, the body cannot eliminate toxins and the toxic burden in our bodies increases. Dehydration can also slow down cellular metabolism and skin cell turnover, which means a slower metabolism and a dull-looking complexion.
- If you get in a 9-1-1 situation where your skin is breaking out before a big event, I recommend for three days drinking only raw smoothies followed by an enema at the end of each day. The enema

will help rid the body more readily of toxic build up in the colon.

If you do this for three days, it may help bring down the inflammation in your skin, which can calm any stubborn outbreaks. Also, while doing this, drink at least fifty fluid ounces of water to help flush out the toxins from your system and take a good probiotic.

- Last, I recommend checking your tongue in the morning upon rising. If you have a white film coating on your tongue, it may be an indicator you have an overgrowth of yeast in the system. If this is the case, a yeast cleanse is recommended.

  Gaia Herbs has wonderful yeast cleanse, which is a three-part system you incorporate with your daily meals for two weeks. I like this program, because it is not too limiting. I find if any detox is too limiting, I will stop after a few days.

Chapter 14

The Spiritual Diva

No book of mine would be complete if I did not talk of my spiritual journey paralleling my quest for an acne-free life. Spirituality is an important part of overall health and can be beneficial to controlling stress and stress-related symptoms that can lead to acne.

I have always been a seeker of knowledge as well as being curious about all the whys in life. I am one of those people who want to know why. Trust me; I have driven a few people crazy!

I suppose this is also why I chose to study philosophy when I was a student at UC Berkeley. I must admit, I left

Berkeley more confused by the meaning and purpose of life than when I entered.

Why is the meaning of life and its associated whys so important to me? I suppose it has to do with the circumstances of my childhood. I was a very sensitive child, exposed to a lot of violence in my home. It had a profound impact on the way I felt about and dealt with the world.

By the time I was a teenager, I was a neurotic mess—this may be an understatement. I was plagued with anxiety and depression, and had difficultly functioning daily.

On more than one occasion I called 9-1-1 because I thought I was having a heart attack. At nineteen years old this may have seemed ridiculous, but while in the midst of a full blown panic attack, this seemed to be a rational conclusion.

At one point in my life, I was so incapacitated by my anxiety I could not drive. I had to temporally drop out of school because I was terrified to travel outside of a few block radius of my house. I had images in my head about having a panic attack in public and dying. I decided it was better to die on my living room floor, so people would not step on my body as they exited the subway train.

I spent years in and out of therapist offices trying to deconstruct the labyrinth in my mind. I desperately wanted to function as normally as possible, so I could lead a life pursuing my dreams and passions. I could not do this experiencing ten or more panic attacks daily. When I was not having panic attacks I was on Xanax, which dulled my drive and passion for life.

For months at a time, I was medicated and felt apathetic, or I was not medicated and on an emotional roller coaster. I would swing from being extremely happy and driven to not wanting to get out of bed.

I remember spending days in bed staring out my window contemplating the worth of living. During such moments, I did not want to eat or communicate with the outside world, I just want to lie in my bed and watch the world pass by me.

In my vibrant moments, I would be an energetic passionate woman who cared about being athletic and healthy. Yet, in my down moments, I would start smoking and not caring about what I put into my body. I remember a moment when I was coming out of a down phase, I ran on my treadmill, and then smoked a cigarette.

I felt compulsive, manic, and completely out-of-control of my life. I kept seeking help, but nothing seemed to help much. I was tired of taking medication that numbed me.

At one point I sought group therapy. I figured if I was in a room with a bunch of people who had similar feelings, I would not feel so isolated.

I have to say group therapy was tremendously helpful for me. The therapists leading the group helped me realize all my panic attacks were a manifestation of my suppressed rage. I spent a year hitting a foam bat against the floor, screaming at all the people who hurt me and tormented my thoughts up to that point in my life.

Then one evening during a therapy session, as I was wailing the bat against the ground, a strange thing happened that started me on the pathway to my new life. I started to cry. I really sobbed. I think I sobbed for over two hours straight because when I finally looked up, every one in my therapy group was gone, but the therapist.

He look at me with a tremendous amount of compassion and said, "Dawn, I think you had a breakthrough tonight."

He stayed with me for a while longer. All this rage that was in me was unbound and I started expressing my hurt, disappointments, and losses. I never forget that night as my therapist walked me to my car in the Stockton/Sutter garage in San Francisco. It was that night when I thought maybe I can be free, maybe I can live the life I wanted to live.

The funny part though was as soon as my rage and panic attacks subsided, was the moment my skin became a natural disaster. Now, I see having bad skin allowed me to hyper focus on something, and it was also a way to hide my true self from the world.

Bad skin days would give me an excuse to self-loathe and limit myself from human interaction and events. I could bury myself in my studies or a book and feel content.

I suppose looking back, this was my way of cycling through highs and lows without seeming too manic. That is, on my good skin days I would be a happy bubbly person, and on my bad skin days I would feel depressed, ugly, and not want to leave the house.

I felt content in this cycle. I would take medication prescribed by the doctor and have clear, irritated skin that could be masked with makeup. Then I did not take the acne medication, self-loathe, and try to find alternative therapies. I traded the up and down feeling of being on and off of Xanax for feeling happy or self-loathing while on and off antibiotics.

I became aware of my patterning and addiction to needing to feel drastic emotional swings in order to feel stable and content. It makes sense now—I was stuck in a pattern of replicating how my life was as a child.

When a person grows up in a house where there is violence and substance abuse, life is a constant roller coaster. One day everything is great and seems okay, and the next everything is completely chaotic.

At the time, I did not realize I replaced panic attacks with Xanax, and then with acne. That is, once I felt like I had control over my panic attacks. I needed something else to give me the emotional up and down I craved. Acne filled that space for me.

When I would oscillate from having acne to clear skin, I would feel intense highs and lows. I would feel great when my skin was doing well, but once I had a bad breakout, I would sink into depression and self-hatred.

Chapter 15

Finding My True Pathway

Being true to me, I started to become completely obsessed with my skin. I became so obsessed with my skin when I finished college I decided to go to school and become an aesthetician. Aside from having my two sons, this is by far the best decision I ever made in my life. I will say that again, becoming an aesthetician was by far the best decision I have ever made in my life!

I was born to be an aesthetician. The day I decided to become an aesthetician is the day I started to live my life to its full potential. If someone told me at the time how the decision to go to aesthetics school would completely alter the pathway of my life, I would not have believed it.

This may sound dorky, but the day I started my classes I fell in love with life; I loved everything about what I was learning. I loved helping people, giving people facials, and making people feel good. I simply loved this profession.

I was so excited to get up in the morning. I was so excited by the friendships I made in class. One classmate is one of my dearest and best friends to this day.

I was, however, still struggling with acne. I remember my father-in-law at the time commenting I was wasting my time because no one was going to take advice from a girl with "shit all over her face."

I did not let his comments discourage me. I trusted that I was finally on the right pathway. Fortunately, with my newfound knowledge of exfoliation, I started to get clearer skin. My skin was still a struggle for me though.

At one point, I started to get discouraged. The words of my father-in-law kept echoing in my head; I started to think maybe he was right. Who was going to want to get skin care advice from a girl who had a face like mine?

Who was going to hire a girl who has zits emerging on her face every other minute?

After completing my state board exams, I hit the pavement looking for a job. It took me a few months, but I finally found a job up the street from my house. Unfortunately, I struggled with the politics that took place in the salon, and left very shortly after I started.

At this point, the economy was spiraling downward; I was completely discouraged. After some careful consideration, I decided it was time to go into business for myself. I figured I had nothing to lose. I could try and I if I fell on my face, well, at least I tried.

I started Skin Logic, an acne treatment center, in February 2009, one of the worst months in the history of the economy. Knowing the economy was bad, I did not bother trying to secure a small business loan, so my only starting capital was a $2,000.00 credit card. To some people, it may have looked like I was chasing an impossible dream, but I figured I had to become really creative.

My chiropractor at the time had a room not being utilized, so I bartered with him and gave him facials in turn for not having to pay rent the first few months I was trying to establish myself. I borrowed a massage table, bought a ten dollar computer cart off Craigslist and used the rest of my capital to buy professional products for treatments and retail items.

I had no clients when I opened Skin Logic; I used social media tools to drive clients through my door. Did it happen overnight—no! If it happened overnight without struggle, my journey and story would be boring.

The first few months were slow for me. I was getting a few clients here and there, but not enough to make a living. I felt discouraged, but took action to better my web presence in hopes that people would find me when doing Google searches for acne treatments in San Jose.

About six months after I opened, my business started to grow at a steady rate. At the same time, the walls of my personal life started tumbling down around me. As my business started to pick up, my marriage was in a state of complete disaster.

My husband at the time had just finished his PhD, and we had two young sons, who were nearly two years old and three years old. The stress of life was putting a strain on our already tumultuous relationship.

Ten months after opening Skin Logic, I decided to leave my marriage. I walked away from a life, which to some seemed idyllic—I had a handsome, educated husband and two beautiful sons. However, inside the walls of my perfect life, I felt completely disconnected.

I would go to work all day feeling happiness and joy. I would come home at night and felt like life was drained from me. I felt like I was back on that familiar emotional pendulum, oscillating from extreme emotional highs to extreme emotional lows.

I was terrified when I left my marriage with two small children and a small business in a rocky economy. Intuitively, I knew I was making the right decision. In my heart I wanted to leave, but I also had two small children; I was so torn.

I was scared of being a single mother. I was scared I was not going to financially make it—hell, I was just scared.

Then one day in September 2009, three months before walking away from my marriage, a small event took place that was going to completely change my life. It was a Monday, so I was not working. I dropped my oldest son off at preschool, and then my youngest son and I went to the park afterwards.

At the park that day, a man came and sat down next to me. He quickly stated he was not trying to hit on me, he just felt compelled to ask me if I had heard of a book by an author named Wayne Dyer.

I replied no, and he suggested I should get it and read it if I had a chance. After my son was done playing at the park, I drove to the bookstore and bought the book he suggested. It was *Meditations for Manifestations* by Dr. Wayne Dyer.

I went home that day and began reading the book, and then listened to the meditation CD included. I have to be honest, I was a little unsure about all this stuff. I mean, I am a philosophical thinker, yet at the same time can be very skeptical.

The premise of this book is: if you project the thoughts of what you want to manifest in your life out into the world, the universe will bring it to you. Being a skeptic, I tested out this theory. I mediated on the universe to give me a sign I should start practicing the principles of this book. I mediated I wanted a sign my life was on the right pathway, and I was making the right decisions personally and professionally.

Well, what happened next is almost unbelievable? If it did not happen to me, I may not believe it. A few days after making my request to the universe, I fell and knocked out my front tooth. I called my dentist, and she told me to immediately come in so she could examine it.

After taking x-rays, my dentist said I had completely broken the tooth from the root; I would need a dental implant. She referred me to a surgeon in Mountain View, California. She acknowledged it was a bit of a drive, but he was the best and I needed to be careful since it was my front tooth.

She sent me directly there with my x-rays in hand. I arrived at the surgeon's office, filled out some paperwork, and waited for him to see me. About ten minutes later, a man opened the door to the waiting area to call me back to see the doctor.

The man, who called me, was the same man who sat down next to me at the park a week earlier, and told me to read the Wayne Dyer book—I was in shock! I knew that moment this was my sign from the universe. I was on the right pathway. I just had a lot of challenges and hurdles to go through to test my newfound faith.

Three months after this event, I was sitting in a small apartment in downtown San Jose. I walked away from my marriage with the clothes on my back and my kids.

I had no energy to fight for anything at this point in my life. I decided putting my energy into my business and children would give me the most happiness in the long run.

I will not lie. The first year was extremely difficult for me. I felt very alone and isolated. My business was still having ups and downs, and I was unsure if I would be able to keep the doors open.

One night, feeling completely emotionally taxed and on the edge, I put my children to bed, and went into my kitchen, sat on the kitchen floor, and began sobbing. I sat crying until about three o'clock in the morning.

I fell asleep on my kitchen floor curled up in a ball, completely emotionally discouraged. I woke up the next morning, got my children dressed, and took them to their nanny at their father's house.

I would usually go straight to the office after dropping them off, but I decided to head back home and collect myself. I was feeling disheveled from having slept so little.

On top of that, I was feeling emotionally and physically drained.

Driving back to my apartment, I kept going over in my head what to do. Should I close Skin Logic's doors and get a job with a steady paycheck, or should I keep trying to build my business for a while longer. I felt confused and scared, and I had dire thoughts of losing my children and being homeless.

By this point, I had been practicing my meditations daily, so I decided before I headed off to work for the day to sit, meditate, and ask the universe for some guidance. Before going into my meditation, I focused on a sign being given to me, so I had confirmation I was doing the right thing by keeping Skin Logic open.

After about forty minutes of meditation, I got up and walked into my kitchen to get some tea. I picked up my cellphone, and there was a new email in the inbox. I opened the email and began reading it.

I could not believe it; there was an email sitting in my inbox from *Skin Inc.* magazine, one of the largest publications in my industry. They wanted to do an article on me! I had to read it about a dozen times to make sure my mind was not playing tricks on me. I received my confirmation all right!

I have read a lot of books about entrepreneurs; these authors always talk about the moment when they know although hurdles and challenges still lie ahead, everything is going to work out. They know the vision they are striving for is going to be attained.

Getting that email from *Skin Inc.* magazine was such a moment for me. I sat there on my living room floor drinking my tea and crying. I knew I was on the right pathway, and I just had to hold my vision no matter what the obstacles.

It was within this moment I decided *no* and *impossible* were no longer going to part of my vocabulary. I also knew in that moment my vision was going to become my life.

I headed off to work that day with a newfound hope and confidence. I started treating and visualizing my business as if it were already successful. I started living my life as if everything I wanted was already right there in front of me. I started imagining what it would feel like to live a life where all my dreams were manifested into reality.

To this day, I still do not deviate from this thought of action. My visions change and grow, but I never stray from the thought my life is not everything it is supposed to be.

I also started giving gratitude for everything in my life. I give gratitude for my children, clients, and future clients. I give gratitude for everything down to the hot water I have when I take my shower in the morning.

On days when I feel down, I walk through the world giving gratitude and being happy for others' successes. If I see a nice car drive by that I admire, I am happy and grateful for that person, who can afford the car.

If I read an article about someone who is achieving success in their business ventures, I am happy and grateful for them. The more I am grateful for others and their abundance, the more abundance I receive.

Trust me, I am far from perfect. I still have my days when I wake up and feel down. I have tools in my toolbox and good skin care to help me lift myself out the doldrums much faster than in the past.

When I am having a hectic day and feeling disheveled, I give myself a time out to go mediate and re-center myself. I allow myself space to feel what is really going on with me. I allow myself to be okay with where I am at during that particular moment.

I give myself permission to be perfectly me. By being perfectly me, I have the space and energy to help others be perfectly themselves.

Also, now I do not look at acne as a disease that has cursed my life; I look at it as a blessing. If I never had acne, I would never be where I am today. Because of acne, I am extremely passionate about health, fitness, and leading a positive and emotionally balanced life.

Acne also led me to my calling in life—being an aesthetician. I feel truly blessed to wake up every morning and have the opportunity to help people like me, who struggle with skin issues. There is truly no better feeling in the world than when a client walks through my door after struggling with acne with clear, glowing skin.

Seriously, sometimes I want to start dancing and doing jumping jacks because I am so happy for them! I feel truly blessed, and yes, I am living a happy and acne-free life!

Sample Daily Menu

Upon rising drink one quart of purified water before juicing, coffee, or tea.

Breakfast: Get Your Glow On Morning Elixir

Snack: Fruit

Mid-Morning: The Most Amazing Smoothie Ever

Lunch: Everything But The Kitchen Sink Alkalinizing Salad

Mid-Afternoon: Chia Seed Pudding

Dinner: Protein and Vegetables

If you are feeling hungry during the day you can eat as much fruit as you wish.

Make sure to drink lots water. Hunger can sometime be a false signal of dehydration.

Day One

Skin Condition: ____________________________________
____
____

Breakfast: ____
____
____

Snack: ____
____
____

Lunch: ____
____
____

Snack: ____
____
____

Dinner: ____
____
____

Daily water intake: _________________________________
____
____

Supplements: _______________________________________
____
____

Day Two

Skin Condition: ______________________________

____

____

Breakfast: ______________________________

____

____

Snack: ______________________________

____

____

Lunch: ______________________________

____

____

Snack: ______________________________

____

____

Dinner: ______________________________

____

____

Daily water intake: ______________________________

____

____

Supplements: ______________________________

____

____

Day Three

Skin Condition: ______________________________________

____

____

Breakfast: ____

____

____

Snack: ____

____

____

Lunch: ____

____

____

Snack: ____

____

____

Dinner: ____

____

____

Daily water intake: ___________________________________

____

____

Supplements: ____

____

____

Day Four

Skin Condition: ______________________________

____

____

Breakfast: ______________________________

____

____

Snack: ______________________________

____

____

Lunch: ______________________________

____

____

Snack: ______________________________

____

____

Dinner: ______________________________

____

____

Daily water intake: ______________________________

____

____

Supplements: ______________________________

____

____

Day Five

Skin Condition: ______________________________
____
____

Breakfast: ___________________________________
____
____

Snack: _______________________________________
____
____

Lunch: _______________________________________
____
____

Snack: _______________________________________
____
____

Dinner: ______________________________________
____
____

Daily water intake: ___________________________
____
____

Supplements: _________________________________
____
____

Day Six

Skin Condition: ________________________________

____

____

Breakfast: ____________________________________

____

____

Snack: ____

____

____

Lunch: ____

____

____

Snack: ____

____

____

Dinner: _______________________________________

____

____

Daily water intake: ____________________________

____

____

Supplements: __________________________________

____

____

Day Seven

Skin Condition: ______________________________
____
____

Breakfast: ___________________________________
____
____

Snack: _______________________________________
____
____

Lunch: _______________________________________
____
____

Snack: _______________________________________
____
____

Dinner: ______________________________________
____
____

Daily water intake: ___________________________
____
____

Supplements: _________________________________
____
____

Day Eight

Skin Condition: ______________________________________
____
____

Breakfast: ____
____
____

Snack: ____
____
____

Lunch: ____
____
____

Snack: ____
____
____

Dinner: ____
____
____

Daily water intake: ___________________________________
____
____

Supplements: ____
____
____

Day Nine

Skin Condition: ______________________________________
____
____

Breakfast: ____
____
____

Snack: ____
____
____

Lunch: ____
____
____

Snack: ____
____
____

Dinner: ____
____
____

Daily water intake: ____________________________________
____
____

Supplements: ____
____
____

Day Ten

Skin Condition: ______________________________________

____

____

Breakfast: ____

____

____

Snack: ____

____

____

Lunch: ____

____

____

Snack: ____

____

____

Dinner: ____

____

____

Daily water intake: ___________________________________

____

____

Supplements: ____

____

____

Day Eleven

Skin Condition: ________________________________

____

____

Breakfast: ____________________________________

____

____

Snack: ______________________________________

____

____

Lunch: ______________________________________

____

____

Snack: ______________________________________

____

____

Dinner: _____________________________________

____

____

Daily water intake: ____________________________

____

____

Supplements: _________________________________

____

____

Day Twelve

Skin Condition: ______________________________
____
____

Breakfast: ___________________________________
____
____

Snack: _______________________________________
____
____

Lunch: _______________________________________
____
____

Snack: _______________________________________
____
____

Dinner: ______________________________________
____
____

Daily water intake: ___________________________
____
____

Supplements: _________________________________
____
____

Day Thirteen

Skin Condition: ____

____

____

Breakfast: ____

____

____

Snack: ____

____

____

Lunch: ____

____

____

Snack: ____

____

____

Dinner: ____

____

____

Daily water intake: ____

____

____

Supplements: ____

____

____

Day Fourteen

Skin Condition: ______________________________

____

____

Breakfast: ___________________________________

____

____

Snack: _______________________________________

____

____

Lunch: _______________________________________

____

____

Snack: _______________________________________

____

____

Dinner: ______________________________________

____

____

Daily water intake: ___________________________

____

____

Supplements: _________________________________

____

____

Day Fifteen

Skin Condition: ______________________________

____

____

Breakfast: ___________________________________

____

____

Snack: _______________________________________

____

____

Lunch: _______________________________________

____

____

Snack: _______________________________________

____

____

Dinner: ______________________________________

____

____

Daily water intake: ___________________________

____

____

Supplements: _________________________________

____

____

Day Sixteen

Skin Condition: ________________________________
____
____

Breakfast: ____________________________________
____
____

Snack: ____
____
____

Lunch: ____
____
____

Snack: ____
____
____

Dinner: _______________________________________
____
____

Daily water intake: ____________________________
____
____

Supplements: __________________________________
____
____

Day Seventeen

Skin Condition: ______________________________________
____
____

Breakfast: ____
____
____

Snack: ____
____
____

Lunch: ____
____
____

Snack: ____
____
____

Dinner: ____
____
____

Daily water intake: ___________________________________
____
____

Supplements: ____
____
____

Day Eighteen

Skin Condition: ____

____

____

Breakfast: ____

____

____

Snack: ____

____

____

Lunch: ____

____

____

Snack: ____

____

____

Dinner: ____

____

____

Daily water intake: ____

____

____

Supplements: ____

____

____

Day Nineteen

Skin Condition: ______________________________

____

____

Breakfast: ___________________________________

____

____

Snack: _______________________________________

____

____

Lunch: _______________________________________

____

____

Snack: _______________________________________

____

____

Dinner: ______________________________________

____

____

Daily water intake: ___________________________

____

____

Supplements: _________________________________

____

____

Day Twenty

Skin Condition: ______________________________
____
____

Breakfast: ______________________________
____
____

Snack: ______________________________
____
____

Lunch: ______________________________
____
____

Snack: ______________________________
____
____

Dinner: ______________________________
____
____

Daily water intake: ______________________________
____
____

Supplements: ______________________________
____
____

Day Twenty-One

Skin Condition: ______________________________
____
____

Breakfast: ______________________________
____
____

Snack: ______________________________
____
____

Lunch: ______________________________
____
____

Snack: ______________________________
____
____

Dinner: ______________________________
____
____

Daily water intake: ______________________________
____
____

Supplements: ______________________________
____
____

Day Twenty-Two

Skin Condition: ______________________________

Breakfast: ______________________________

Snack: ______________________________

Lunch: ______________________________

Snack: ______________________________

Dinner: ______________________________

Daily water intake: ______________________________

Supplements: ______________________________

Day Twenty-Three

Skin Condition: ______________________________
____
____

Breakfast: ___________________________________
____
____

Snack: _______________________________________
____
____

Lunch: _______________________________________
____
____

Snack: _______________________________________
____
____

Dinner: ______________________________________
____
____

Daily water intake: ___________________________
____
____

Supplements: _________________________________
____
____

Day Twenty-Four

Skin Condition: ______________________________________

____

____

Breakfast: ____

____

____

Snack: ____

____

____

Lunch: ____

____

____

Snack: ____

____

____

Dinner: ____

____

____

Daily water intake: ___________________________________

____

____

Supplements: ____

____

____

Day Twenty-Five

Skin Condition: ____________________________________

____

____

Breakfast: ____

____

____

Snack: ____

____

____

Lunch: ____

____

____

Snack: ____

____

____

Dinner: ____

____

____

Daily water intake: _________________________________

____

____

Supplements: _______________________________________

____

____

Day Twenty-Six

Skin Condition: ____________________________________

____

____

Breakfast: ____

____

____

Snack: ____

____

____

Lunch: ____

____

____

Snack: ____

____

____

Dinner: ____

____

____

Daily water intake: _________________________________

____

____

Supplements: _____________________________________

____

____

Day Twenty-Seven

Skin Condition: ____

____

____

Breakfast: ____

____

____

Snack: ____

____

____

Lunch: ____

____

____

Snack: ____

____

____

Dinner: ____

____

____

Daily water intake: ____

____

____

Supplements: ____

____

____

Day Twenty-Eight

Skin Condition: ____________________________________
____
____

Breakfast: ____________________________________
____
____

Snack: ____________________________________
____
____

Lunch: ____________________________________
____
____

Snack: ____________________________________
____
____

Dinner: ____________________________________
____
____

Daily water intake: ____________________________________
____
____

Supplements: ____________________________________
____
____

About the Author

Dawn Amador holds a bachelor's degree in analytic philosophy from the University of California Berkeley. She also attended the graduate school at San Francisco's Academy of Art University (AAU) where she studied product development and manufacturing.

During her studies at UC Berkeley and AAU, she struggled with acne issues, and her passion for skin care and nutrition grew. It was during this time when Amador started to consider how she could combine her passions for education, research, and product development to help others who struggled with similar skin issues. After starting graduate school, she decided to switch directions and obtain her aesthetician license and open an acne treatment center.

In February 2009, Amador opened up Skin Logic with no clients, a borrowed massage table, a smartphone and a laptop. She only had five products in her back bar and was selling retail out of a desk drawer.

Today Skin Logic has a customer base of over 1,000 and has never created a printed menu, let alone marketed through print advertising. Skin Logic grew using with minimal overhead and social media tools such as Google Analytics, Yelp, blogs, and *BookFresh* to drive clientele to its website and services 24/7.

Amador also took a non-traditional approach to treating acne by looking at acne as a systemic issue as well as a topical one. She coaches her clients on health and wellness and treats acne with organic ingredients versus the traditional model of harsh chemicals. Taking this approach leads to long-term solutions, which help achieve internal balance as well as beautiful glowing skin.